TRIUMPH OVER **LUNG** DISEASE

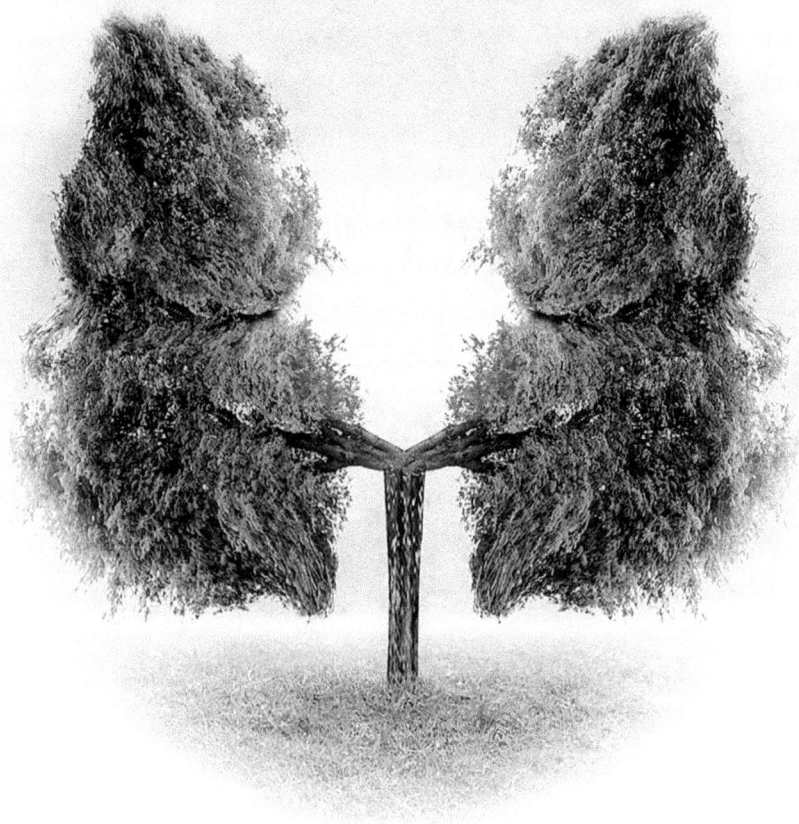

*How to Regain **Breath** and **Vitality***

LESSONS LEARNED FROM HEROES

TRIUMPH
OVER
LUNG
DISEASE

MARILYN KLINGLER RN, BS, M.ED.

MANY**SEASONS**PRESS

Mesa, Arizona • 2020

FIRST EDITION

Triumph Over Lung Disease, How to Regain Breath and Vitality

Contact the author at: TriumphToolkit@gmail.com

A percentage of proceeds from this book will support non-profit organizations promoting COPD education and research.

Published by Many Seasons Press
(An Imprint of MultimediaPublishingProject.com)
PO Box 50553
Mesa, AZ 85208
480.939.9689 | ManySeasonsPress.com

Cover & book interior designed by Yolie Hernandez
(AZBookDesigner@icloud.com)

Cover art by Cinemanikor (Shutterstock ID: 1543378691)

Author photo by Carley Barton

ISBN 13: 978-1-936885-35-0

Disclaimer: This book is not a medical book but an opportunity to share ideas, tools, and inspiration.

Names and stories in this book are composites, built from pulmonary rehabilitation experiences that I have witnessed or that have been shared with me. They do not reflect any specific individuals.

This book is dedicated to all the men and women with Lung Disease who dared to live life to the fullest.

It is not the years in your life but the life in your years that counts.

—Adlai Stevenson

Table of Contents

Acknowledgements

Behind every author are hours of supporting work by caring colleagues and friends. Heartfelt thanks to my publisher, Yolie Hernandez (ManySeasonsPress.com) and editor Maryann Waugh for their great ideas and attention to details. My sincere gratitude to my friend and colleague, Stephanie Barton who worked closely with me, page by page to make this book happen. I am so grateful to author Lee Simonich for sharing her proficiency in writing and encouraging me on, fine tuning the details. Special thanks to pulmonologist, Dr. Slobig for his wisdom and encouragement over the years and who taught me to see the whole patient, not just the disease. Many thanks also to John and Connie, James, Dennis and Nancy. I so appreciate the much-needed support and suggestions provided by my husband, Larry. Thanks to so many who shared their stories and their insights, who helped and supported me on this journey of discovery and expression.

Foreword

I am a pulmonary nurse. I am the conduit for what needs to be shared with you and I am humbled by the people from whom I have learned. Synchronicity is defined as "the coincidental occurrence of events...that seem related but are not explained by conventional mechanisms of causality. This book, *Triumph Over Lung Disease: How to Regain Breath and Vitality*, initially started over 6 years ago, was stuffed in a back file labeled 'who knows, maybe someday.'

But have you ever noticed in your life how synchronicity plays out when least expected? There is a reason why this book is being completed and released now.

Just as this book was being submitted to the publisher for printing the COVID-19 pandemic erupted and life radically changed for us all. So many innocent victims were succumbing to this deadly respiratory virus. While waiting for the printed first edition, I realized that the book was not finished.

How can I best support those already coping with lung disease to stay healthy and also those who for the first time are confronting post COVID-19 lung damage?

COVID-19 needed to be addressed in clear and practical terms. Studies, strategies, insights from professionals, and those with first-hand experience of the disease needed to be gathered and reviewed. How can you best protect yourself? What happens if I do get sick? And what happens after?

At the end of the book, I have included a final chapter focusing on COVID-19 prevention, survival, and recuperation. The tools and strategies there and in this book will guide your journey through the turbid waters of the COVID-19 pandemic.

1

Why This Book?

You have changed me- opened my heart and mind to the possibilities.

When crisis occurs, it is normal to feel angry or emotionally numb. The world you knew has disappeared. You are forced to fall back, regroup and figure out how to cope. How do you move forward with this albatross that stunts your energy and your breath? The transition towards a new forward-facing identity takes patience and persistence. It means finding and engaging those inner and outer resources. How open are you to new ways of thinking, new ways of doing things? You may find that the things that bring meaning and purpose in your life change as you grow. Are you ready to move forward? Your choice.

We are born, we die: that's the cycle of life. Even the Sequoia, standing tall and silent for thousands of years, able to fend off the ravages of fire, eventually dies. Our bodies recycle into fodder for nature to absorb and recycle.

So, my point is to use what time we have between these two events, wisely, however we choose. Some choose to explore the world's wonders, amass great amounts of money, create monuments, or become the best of something. Others choose to make a difference. We all choose a track, whether we do it intentionally or it just happens to us. I suspect its roots lie in our subconscious personality. And whatever track we choose, it is not without plenty of obstacles.

I am a nurse. According to recent polls I am a member of the most trusted profession in the country. I've worked in most specialties in and out of hospitals, ICU, Tele, Pulmonary, and Emergency. I've taught in schools and universities. Short, blonde and 108 pounds, I can lift and pull with the best of them, respond quickly in emergencies, and at the same time, show compassion. I have administered all sorts of medications and treatments, advised physicians, and assisted in multiple surgical procedures. In that time, I have learned a few things about what it really means to be healthy, how to get healthy and how to stay healthy. A lot of it isn't rocket science and maybe that's why we miss it, because we expect it to be more complicated. But, as the old Indian medicine women profess, 'for every ailment of man, nature has provided a cure.'

Maybe that's why life led me to Pulmonary Rehab. And in doing this I learned about heroes.

Being a hero might best be described as someone who demonstrates courage beyond what's expected, overcoming huge obstacles to make life better for himself and others. A hero makes a difference. A hero is someone like you, someone who cares.

There is a hero within each one of us. We just need to not be afraid to succeed. We have all faced down innumerable challenges in our lives. Some greater than others and here we are. You can and will be a hero again, if you choose.

There are lots of different kinds of challenges in life. Those that we create, and those that we find ourselves confronted with. How many of your greatest challenges were those based on fear and worry? Overcoming the fear and the worry sometimes is the hardest part.

> *"Courage is not the absence of fear, but the triumph over it."* —Nelson Mandela

You have so much more potential than you realize! I see that potential become reality in pulmonary rehab every day as people transform themselves from victims to victors.

Did you ever notice that your greatest achievements were earned primarily with attitude? You made the decision and you decided that you were going to do it! Moving forward just might take a bit of work, and a lot of attitude. We, in pulmonary rehab, the pulmonologist, the nurse, the respiratory therapist, and the exercise physiologist, we will be there with you every step of the way.

We are the cheering squad, the coaches, and the educators. We remind you that life is far from over; and that although life has thrown you a curveball, this curveball has directed you into a new outlook, a new way of connecting and of appreciating the real joys of life. That doesn't happen overnight. Just like the ballplayer, you practice and eventually you get the hit.

Maybe it's a single but you pushed the team closer to a win and they are cheering!

It doesn't mean you are out of the marathon, when you are diagnosed with lung disease, it simply suggests that maybe life isn't all about coming in first and fastest.

As a pulmonary rehab nurse, I have witnessed clients arriving on their first day in a wheelchair, depressed, despondent and weak. After 20 sessions, these same people are up on their feet, walking with confidence and new hope. I have witnessed clients apprehensively entering the gym for the first time, dragging their purse and their portable oxygen, feeling exhausted and short of breath. Upon completing the program, there's pep in their step, and a renewed love of living and being. They have learned how to take the reins of control over their health. They have become part of a community of like-minded friends with a team that cares about them. They are empowered.

Men and women diagnosed with chronic lung disease gain energy and resume a dynamic and connected life. Some go back to work, others resume bicycling or golf; others take up new activities like car mechanics, fishing, writing, painting or Tai Chi. Some knit hats for hospital preemie newborns and still others play trumpet in the band. Many travel to weddings and family birthdays across the country, with and without oxygen. They regain their hope, their confidence and their independence. They worked for those gains though, and they continue to work.

They achieved their goals, and they did it together with supportive team members. But first they had to create their toolkit, they had to learn what really mattered to them, and what their goals were.

Any reconstruction project requires specific tools, depending on the job. This is a toolkit, complete with strategies and information to put your life back together. You will discover that these tools will help to make life a lot easier and a lot clearer.

This is not a medical book, nor does it take the place of your doctor's advice. It is a book that describes the experiences of patients who have faced and taken control over their pulmonary disease utilizing tools and strategies shared along the way. After 10 years of working with clients with all sorts of chronic lung issues, I feel that their stories need to be told and those who are facing lung challenges need to hear them. From these stories you will find hope.

You will be asked to look at yourself, your strengths and your possibilities. I challenge you to look closely, ask yourself the tough questions, and choose to move forward. The questions at the end of each chapter provide the direction. Simply consider and write down your answers. You can and will find the hero inside.

If you have been diagnosed with chronic lung disease, it may have occurred after a crisis, like Joe. Joe is a composite of the many I have worked with over the years. This book will follow Joe from crisis to triumph. Joe, like the others in this book, hit the pit, regrouped, and picked himself back up. In that process, he found himself a better man, a better husband, a better friend; Joe found life to be a much more rewarding and exciting experience, full of gifts and wonders he never noticed before.

You will share in the tragedies and triumphs of men and women, young and old who have regained their hope and discovered their potential.

Life promises change. It's how you deal with these changes that makes the difference. You can perceive them as either disasters or opportunities, punishments or blessings. More than one of my clients recognized their journey as a walk-up call to what really mattered.

My hope is that you will begin the work of finding that blessing in the midst of the storm.

• • •

Take a moment to write down your answers to these questions:

How satisfied are you with your life right now?

_____

_____

_____

_____

Who do you most admire and why?

_____

_____

_____

_____

How might your life be better?

_____

_____

_____

_____

2

Joe: The Upheaval

You believed in me and supported me through difficult times.

J oe and Ellie were getting excited about finally retiring next year, and plunging into that long bucket list of cruises and tours they had been dreaming about for so long. Joe, who loved to fish when he had a free afternoon, imagined himself catching huge salmon in a catamaran sailing vessel off the coast of Alaska. Ellie dreamed of swimming under the waterfalls in Kauai. So, next spring, they were going. They sent the down payment for a three-week, all-inclusive cruise to the islands. 'The salmon fishing could wait until next year', Joe conceded. They would finally have time to relax, be together and have fun. "Eight more months." Joe was thinking. "How am I ever going to be ready to retire? So much is happening at work, it never slows down anymore. I just can't disappoint Ell again. She's had to put up with me all these years. She deserves a medal."

Being VP of sales comes with a lot of headaches, long hours, and broken family plans. It was tough on his family sometimes. But Joe was the dependable one at work; when there was a crisis, he would be the one who always got it done. He was that way at home too. He played by the rules, worked hard. Never missed work.

It was turning into another sixty-hour week, when he started feeling a little run down. "Hey Chuck, we need to follow up on the hardware for the AE2 series. Customer wants it before the… before… the… holiday. Joe looked grey and his tone was chopped, as if he was gasping for air. "Are you doing OK, Joe?" Asked Chuck, "You don't look so good." Joe gripped his chest. "I can't get my…breath…" stammered Joe. Chuck called 911 as Joe slipped into unconsciousness.

Joe awoke to the constant hiss and groan of the ventilator, the blip of the monitor overhead, and a horrible scratching feeling in his throat. The last thing he remembered he was complaining to Chuck that he couldn't breathe. "Where am I?" He thought. He couldn't move. He couldn't feel anything except an overwhelming exhaustion. His eyes narrowed as he looked around; white walls, screens, monitors and machines surrounded him. Tubes, wires and lines tethered him to the bed. "Ellie!', he screamed in his thoughts "Where are you? What's going on? Ellie!" He wanted to yell out but he couldn't; nothing came out. He tried to flail his arms, desperate to wake up from this nightmare, but they felt so heavy. He was petrified. With the breathing tube down his throat, Joe felt paralyzed and numb, unable to even turn his head. He tried to call out, "Hey! Help me someone!" But he couldn't speak, not a sound.

As he lay there in the sterile environment, a gush of anger rose from his belly. He was trapped. He wanted to burn down this place, these sterile walls. He wanted to lash out at these sterile people, at God. "It's not fair! I don't deserve this! I have so much to do." But he was tired, so tired.

He turned his gaze to see Ellie, sitting beside him, gripping his hand. Her face was framed in a luminescent halo under the glow of the overhead lighting. For a few moments, Joe was sure that he was holding hands with an angel and he became calm. She looked into his eyes and smiled. She knew what he was thinking. She and Joe had been together a long time, and she could read his thoughts just from looking at his face.

"Remember that night we got stuck in that freezing cold snowstorm in Colorado, in the mountains, Joe? It was coming down so fast we couldn't see an inch in front of us and there was no one, no one on that narrow winding road. I was so scared I thought that we would both freeze to death that night, or fall off the cliff. You said to me, 'hang on, Ell, we'll get out of this one; takes a helluva lot more to stop us than this'. And inch by inch, slowly but surely, you stayed on that road, and you got us back to the hotel. You have a lot of guts, Joe, and you never gave up. You stuck with it, just like you will this time."

Ellie's eyes, bright and strong, seemed to pierce right into his soul. Joe nodded, remembering that night. He never did share with her how terrified he had felt. But he had maintained his control and moved forward. He needed to protect her; he had to take care of her. What else could he do. "I'm strong,' he thought, 'bullheaded, sometimes, but you're right, Ell. I didn't give up." He looked at her and smiled with his weary eyes. He wanted so much to touch her, tell her "It's okay. I get it. Okay. I can do this, one step at a time." Tears welled up in his eyes. He wasn't feeling that strong, but damned if he would let her know. "I love you so much, Ell." He tried so hard to transfer his thoughts from his mind to hers. Ellie smiled and nodded." I know, Joe. I know. I'm with you every step of the way."

A week later, Joe finally was able to breathe well enough on his own and the tube in his throat was removed. How freeing to be able to breathe, with only a small oxygen canula wrapped around his ears and across his nose. The oxygen that flowed through the canula kept his oxygen numbers up as he started sitting up and moving about a little on his own. He was still incredibly weak and slept most of the day, but he could talk and even eat a little, though he had no appetite and his throat was sore from the tube. It was when he was transferred out of the intensive care unit that he finally sighed with relief. He felt victorious. With Ellie's support and with perseverance, he was going to make it. "I can probably get back to work next week; there's so much to do," he said, "and our cruise is getting closer. I've got to work on getting some strength back. I told you that I wouldn't let you down again." Ellie could see his mind churning and smiled. "There's time Joe, there's plenty of time." He chuckled to himself, "She knows me so well." He thought. He would continue for now, taking it one step at a time.

Dr. Evans, who had monitored Joe's daily progress, arrived one morning as Ellie and Joe were finishing their coffee. Now that Joe was stronger, thinking more clearly, it seemed a good time to discuss the situation.

"Joe, you had a case of acute interstitial pneumonia that almost killed you. You are tough though, and you made it through. But you have some serious scarring in your lungs, I'm afraid. And it's permanent. There's no cure. I'm sorry. You will need to keep on continuous supplemental oxygen to keep your body adequately oxygenated, and you'll be taking daily medications and treatments. You will have good days and not so good days. Take each day as it comes and make the most of it. I'm discharging you. Go home, take your medications and enjoy the rest of your life."

Joe was discharged home in a wheelchair. Joe felt beaten.

• • •

When Joe returned home, he didn't smile anymore. He didn't laugh, and he didn't go back to work. He had lost a lot of weight and his once tall, trim figure was gaunt and bent. Friends and family tried reconnecting with him but it was as if he just wasn't there anymore. He mostly slept, ate little and watched sports on TV. "I let her down again," he kept musing, over and over again. "And now this is what she gets, an invalid." Ellie did what she could to motivate him, to cheer him up. She had even tried to remind him of his silly jokes. After more than two months at home, Ellie got fed up. "Joe, you cannot, I will not let you, give up. You are here, you are alive, and we need to move forward. We are going down to the medical center tomorrow to learn about the rehab program Dr. Evans mentioned at our last appointment."

• • •

Take a moment to write down your answers to these questions:

What was the most difficult challenge that you have faced in your life?

_____

_____

_____

_____

How did you overcome or adapt to this challenge?

_____

_____

_____

What would you tell Joe to help him through this difficult time?

_____

_____

_____

_____

3

Finding the Desire by Finding Yourself

You give us back our hope, when it had been lost.

Brenda had organized a trip to Paris in August with her granddaughter, Sarah. It was a graduation present, just the two of them. They had always been close, and Brenda had promised Sarah the trip a year ago. She and Sarah had planned out every detail. That was before she had suffered a COPD flare up. The doctor called it 'an exacerbation'. It had kept her in the hospital for two weeks. Now she was on continuous oxygen and she simply did not have the breath or the stamina to do much of anything anymore.

Brenda had always been a walker. Every day, she would walk a mile, primarily for her health but also because it made her slow down and appreciate the mornings, the sunshine, and the gardens. She was a bit heavyset with an attractive elegance about her. She had struggled most of her life with her weight. "Big boned, but healthy," the doctor would say. "Don't worry, be happy with who you are."

When Brenda returned home from her recent hospitalization, she felt exhausted. She was using her oxygen continuously and had to increase it when she stood up to do anything. After two months, she had expected to begin feeling like herself again, but not this time. Everything seemed to take so much more effort. She just couldn't seem to bounce back. The trip to Paris was barely three months away.

She was distraught when she started at pulmonary rehab wondering how she would ever handle walking across the large public garden at the Louvre. But Brenda did not want to have to use a wheelchair. Though she assumed her walking days were pretty much over, she was determined to make *that* walk. It was her goal. She had always seen herself as a pretty determined person once she decided on something, but she was losing hope. When she started rehab, she could barely walk for 90 seconds on the treadmill at 0.7 mph without becoming out of breath. "How will I ever make it across that huge courtyard? How will I manage?" She sighed. But, little by little she improved. Gradually, over several weeks, her time on the treadmill increased, and after 12 weeks she was up to 12 minutes.

Brenda's trip was rapidly approaching. She was still worried, but the team had confidence in her. Even her friends there, the other clients in her class, encouraged her. 'Do or do not; there is no try', Yoda had said. Yes. She would do! "Stay calm, breathe, go slow, smile," she kept reminding herself, using the constant refrain of the pulmonary rehab team.

Brenda returned from her visit to Paris, elated, reporting that she had done it. She had strolled across the public garden holding hands with her 17-year-old granddaughter, Sarah. She had walked all the way, right to the steps of the Louvre. When Brenda told us about her trip, she was beaming like a lighthouse; her smile was bigger than her face. "We stopped a few times, just to enjoy the view, she laughed, "and Sarah carried my oxygen for me which helped a lot." Brenda was a hero. She faced her fears, and with the support of her granddaughter, taking slow steps, she made it! It hadn't been easy, but she just remembered to stay calm. She did pursed lip breathing, stopped when she needed to, "and..." she said, "I smiled the entire way." She was proud of herself. She realized that if she could do this, she could do more.

Brenda returned to finish her classes in pulmonary rehab, sharing her success stories with the new members in her class, motivating them to keep working. If she could accomplish so much, they, and you, can too.

Brenda resumed walking each morning at home, small walks, keeping track of her breathing and her oxygen levels. Some days were better than others. But overall, she found that her walks, and her life got a little easier.

Despite the universal illusion of the single warrior destroying the beast and saving the world, the hero does not accomplish great things alone. You are not in this alone. We all support each other. And by supporting each other, we help ourselves.

But, all the support in the world cannot make you change. It cannot do the walk. You are still the one who has to choose that goal and carry it out. How do you unlock that strength that makes some people able to move mountains? - One step at a time. That first step is the most important; it starts you moving. And with each step forward, you are closer to the summit. How do you connect with your inner power? One simple step at a time.

Neil Armstrong took the first step on the moon, but it didn't happen overnight. It took a lot of preparation and hard work by him and thousands of others.

We all dance to a different drum beat. The rate at which we grow and change is unique. And sometimes, we get stuck in the muck and feel paralyzed, unable to make a decision.

How do you start? Discovering your core is good way to start. Are you ready?

Take a moment to write down your answers to these questions:

What do you like most about yourself?

_____

_____

_____

What engages you?

_____

_____

_____

What are you most proud of?

_____

_____

_____

What are you afraid of?

_____

_____

_____

4

The Greatest Achievement

You open the way for us to move forward, redesign our thinking.

Be brave. Lung disease brings changes. Your job is to adapt to the changes in the best ways possible. It's not always easy. You have to find the stamina to pick yourself back up when you fall down.

Ken arrived in a wheelchair for his preliminary assessment and orientation. He explained that he required a therapist to work with him at his home as he would be unable to walk and lacked the stamina to travel to outpatient rehab. His caregiver, Nancy, agreed. "He is not strong enough, he has severe lung disease," she said. I nod my head in understanding and compassion. "You are here," I explain, "You are ready. You see, pulmonary rehab is more than a series of exercises, it involves not only strengthening the body, but the spirit and the mind as well. You need to understand that this is not a lone climb up Mount Everest, but a group activity. You don't do this on your own, try it for few weeks and see how it works out."

With effort, Ken began attending twice weekly sessions, building his strength and stamina on the NuStep. After three weeks, he was on the treadmill, despite my trepidation. I wasn't sure if he was really ready for it. He was insistent and it was hard to say no. He climbed onto the treadmill, applied his safety clip, took a breath and turned it on. Ken walked at 0.6mph for one minute, with me by his side, ready to catch him or stop the machine if he showed any trouble. But he did it! And his oxygen numbers stayed within range. We were both beaming with joy. "Looking good!", one of the other's yelled. Ken could not have been prouder. He continued forward from there, every day, little by little with thirty-second increases each week.

Funny, that's how it starts, that one minute, or maybe it's only thirty seconds. Once you accomplish what may seem like such a small thing, you find you can do it; and you want to do more.

Ken was energized. That energizing feeling seemed to diffuse into his attitude and his personality in the gym. He became brighter, more expressive, and more confident. He had hope. He was motivated.

Ken continued to improve, walking a little longer and a little faster, maintaining his oxygen levels and feeling better and better. Some days were great; some days were not so great. Sometimes, he had setbacks and couldn't do the treadmill. "That's OK, some days that just happens, you'll do better next time," I said. "Listen to your body." By his twentieth session, Ken was walking into rehab with his cane, pulling his oxygen behind him, grinning from ear to ear. He was still using oxygen, but he was now armed with the confidence that, with effort, and support, he could accomplish things on his own.

It's not the marathon runner who improves his time by 30 seconds that is most admirable, but the person in the wheelchair who gets up to take his first step. The smallest step becomes the greatest achievement.

Harrison Ford, in the movie, "Henry" plays an arrogant Wall Street tycoon who suffers a brain trauma causing paralysis. Although physicians warned him that he would not walk again, Henry would not give in. After months of struggle, he takes his first few steps on the parallel bars with his physical therapist close by. Tears of joy wash down his face. There had been no triumph in his entire life as momentous as this.

The everyday heroes in pulmonary rehab used to be just like Joe. They believed in the negative prognosis and stopped trying. They had no stamina, no confidence, and no toolbox. After rehab, they discovered their power. Like Henry, like Ken, they decided to go for it, gaining the strength and the knowledge to carry on, adapting as they needed to. They found the tools.

They don't spend their time worrying anymore that their oxygen supply could run out before reaching home. They know that they have planned, prepared, and that they are fine. Sometimes, it still takes deliberate effort just to get out of bed in the morning, but they do it, and it gets better. They check in with themselves and recognize if it's just 'one of those days' and they carry on either way.

The despair of feeling like a dependent, a victim, has been replaced with an understanding of their potential and of their present limits. Everyone has limits. That doesn't mean that they are etched in stone. You have the choice to stretch limits in smart ways, using the tools you'll soon learn.

. . .

Take a moment to write down your answers to these questions:

How would you like to see yourself a year from now? Describe yourself.

_____

_____

_____

_____

What part of this picture of yourself is the most important and why?

_____

_____

_____

_____

What could be your first step towards achieving this picture?

_____

_____

_____

_____

5

Joe: Getting Acquainted with Hope

You share the light of life with everyone you touch.

Ellie and Joe sat apprehensively in the small conference room. Waiting. Joe's concentrator was turned off and his canula was now attached to a green oxygen tank on wheels. They were distracted by the conversations of other people laughing and chatting and the hum of equipment in the gym across the hall. Joe thought, "What am I doing here? All that work, making this appointment, driving here, filling out forms, and for what? There is no way in hell I can even begin to go back to a gym! This place is not for me. Why, damn it, did Dr. Evans even think that this might be an option. He is dreaming! I just want to go home." Joe's head dropped into his hands as he sat. "Ellie," Joe said. "We should …."

Sandy, the exercise physiologist who had just reviewed Joe's paperwork, arrived and greeted them. "I'm so happy that you are coming to Pulmonary Rehab, Joe. Looks like you have been dealing with a lot this past year. It's been difficult, I imagine." Joe relaxed. "Okay," he thought, "she gets it; it has been bad." But his negative thoughts continued. "My life is over... just surviving day-to-day... even my relationship with Ellie has been rough.... I can't do this rehab thing..."

Tall, slim with long straight auburn hair, Sandy looked at Joe with understanding. "How are you doing?" "Fine," says Joe. He knew that she knew he was just not in the mood. "Let's focus on how you would like to be feeling." Ellie said nothing; she simply sat next to Joe and listened. "Tell me what you are doing now for your regular daily activities. What do you do for fun; what are your hobbies?"

Sandy listened as Joe shared his daily routine, "I wake up at 10 usually, I don't sleep very well. I sit on the side of the bed and I take my inhalers. That takes fifteen to twenty minutes. Sometimes I shower, but most days, I don't bother. Then, I have breakfast, coffee. Then I go to my 'king chair', my Lazy Boy, and settle in for my shows. "Jeopardy," "Price is Right," "What's my Line," "Wheel of Fortune," then Sports......Saying all this out loud Joe realized that he had not been doing much at all. Sandy simply nodded. Ellie brings me my snacks and gets my nebulizer. I just don't have much energy. He felt like someone, at last, was truly hearing him, that someone truly understood. He could see the light of understanding on Sandy's face. "Maybe, she might have some ideas for me," he started to hope.

"As you can see, there is a gym with lots of different machines that can help you eventually regain your strength and your stamina. You might be intimidated by that right now. You see, some of your fatigue and shortness of breath may be due to your lung problem. Some of it is simply a loss of muscle tissue from not moving much over the past several months. It also might be from your state of mind which, maybe, is not too optimistic right now."

Sandy checked his oxygen gauge. "Two liters, okay." She then took his blood pressure and his oximetry. "126/78, and 94%. Good. I'm going to ask you to walk, and I'm going to time your walk for six minutes. If you need to stop and rest, that's fine. If you walk for a minute and say you are done, that's okay. Just do the best you can. This is a starting point to measure where you are right now as compared to where you will be after you complete the program. It also helps me gauge your exercise prescription."

Joe struggled up out his wheelchair as Ellie pulled under his arm to help. He started walking down the hall, pulling the green oxygen tank behind him, "Just follow those foot tracks on the floor." Sandy guided him. He walked through the gym, noticing the number of people, working out on the machines, smiling, talking. Joe walked, one foot after the other, slowly, deliberately, grabbing the wall at times to keep from faltering. He walked for almost two minutes before he had to rest. It usually took him less than a minute to walk from his lazy boy to the bathroom which he did maybe five times a day. Six minutes had sounded like nothing, but wow, that was a long time! He was getting tuckered out fast. Joe remembered how he used to sprint through the park on Saturdays, three miles nonstop, just a couple of years before. "Another time, another life," he thought. He walked another minute and stopped to rest again. Finally, after another 30 seconds. He was exhausted. "I'm done."

"Good job." Sandy said, after taking his vital signs one more time. "Your oxygen numbers stayed up in the normal range and you walked 500 feet! I can see that you have potential, Joe. You can and will get stronger. Your muscles will remember. I'm looking forward to that six-minute walk at the end of the program, when I will measure you again. You will find it a whole lot easier! Your muscles are weak now and you tend to try to rush too much. I want to get you on the treadmill, slowly at first and we'll build you up, gradually. I'm excited for you!"

Sandy's enthusiasm and her belief in his ability to get better was like an elixir for Ellie and Joe. Joe was a little afraid to believe her, but she looked so sincere and she should know, she's been doing this for, what did she say, the last six years?

"Before you leave today, I want to give you a homework assignment. I saw you walk for two minutes today. I want you to walk twice, every day at home, for one and a half minutes. A little slower please, and stop if you want, but do it twice a day. This is not a race. Can you do it?" Joe nodded. "Okay, then after one week, I want you to increase that time by a half a minute. That's it. You will do great, Joe. Keep up that 'stick to it' attitude, be consistent, even if you have to push yourself a bit. Just get here, twice a week at 11: am. Promise?" Joe nodded. "I'll be looking forward to working with you." She said, beaming.

Joe and Ellie walked out of the center, both smiling and feeling that there was hope. "She sure seemed to know her stuff," said Joe. "I like her." "I do too," said Ellie.

• • •

Take a moment to write down your answers to these questions:

What would it take to make you move forward?

_____

_____

_____

_____

What is holding you back?

_____

_____

_____

_____

Where, or from whom, do you get your strength?

_____

_____

_____

_____

6

The Inside Story

You make great things happen in little ways.

Y ou are a continuous miracle. With your first moment of life, you inspired life itself. The air you breathe, with each inhalation, helps create the person you are becoming. It connects us to all of life. That air continues to be breathed in and out, by trillions of life forms, changing, and being used, again and again, to create more life and more experience. Have you ever taken a moment to connect with your own breath? Experience, now for a moment the flow of oxygen from your nostrils down your windpipe into your lungs. Feel it being absorbed into your bloodstream and transported throughout your entire system to each cell. This oxygen is being provided to each cell continuously so it can survive for you to enjoy and experience, function and grow.

Did you know each cell has enough oxygen stored for only four seconds? After that, it will begin to die. Yet, they continue their tasks, never giving a single thought, a single worried moment to the idea that the next delivery of oxygen might not be coming in time. Cells don't worry about the future. They are too engaged in the present.

We might listen to the cells in our body. Each of these trillions of cells carry out the tasks of survival, working in community with other cells. Groups of different functioning cells are constantly communicating and cooperating, integrating into the whole. As lone cells, they cannot survive on their own.

Working together towards a balanced and harmonious body allows a balanced and harmonious cell to exist.

The cell is a single organism yet lives in an interdependent community of cells, tissues, and organs. The intuitive wisdom of these cells, to heal, to grow and adapt, and balance is a more complex system of mechanics than we could ever in our conscious mind handle ourselves for a single moment: managing and responding to invading germs, changing temperatures, balancing acidity levels, producing energy, ingesting and digesting, absorbing and utilizing oxygen for energy, reproducing, eliminating waste, healing and growing. The list continues. The single cell is incredibly efficient, quick thinking, and resourceful, a true spark of genius.

We are exactly like each single cell, capable of so much on our own, but part of a bigger system, critical to our ability to thrive. We are built to love and be loved, to exist in an interdependent social system, to adapt to life's changes. We are equipped with incredible intuitive wisdom, *(if we listen) t*o heal.

Spend some time connecting with your cells, your organs, your body. Appreciate for a moment what your body accomplishes for you. Interestingly, we never think about the well-functioning machinery of our bodies until it gives us a problem. Teachers, parents, and managers recognize that when we are stroked with appreciative responses to our actions, we are much more likely to continue to try harder to live up to expectations and do more. If we are continually criticized and put down, we become more and more demoralized, depressed, and tired. Did you ever consider the thought that your lungs can hear you when you are talking about them? Are you appreciating or criticizing? Are your lungs "bad" or are they doing the best they can?

There was a journalist who was doing research for a story on psychics for his upcoming journal article. He had been having some trouble with his back recently and had become frustrated and angry, complaining to friends and family about this chronic pain. He was so angry that his 'bad back' kept him from doing the things he wanted to do. When he arrived to interview the psychic, she immediately confronted him. "Have you been yelling at your back? Have you been saying negative things about your back? Your back is simply doing what your words express! It assumes you expect a bad back and its working hard to meet your expectations!" The journalist had never met this person before but recognized that she was accurately reading his body.

Japanese scientist Masaru Emoto discovered that when highly charged words are expressed in water, the water crystallizes into certain patterns when allowed to freeze. Anger, frustration, and hostility are expressed as distorted ugly crystals whereas positive emotions of compassion, love, and joy are expressed in the frozen water as beautifully formed crystals.

As our bodies are made up primarily of water, 65%, your anger and frustration can be expressed physically in your body. So, what are you saying to and about your body? Research has shown again and again that we live up to expectations. What type of crystals are being created inside your cells, inside your body?

The principal of a very large grade school met with two of his teachers prior to the beginning of the school year and notified them that they would have a class made up of the highest performing students in the state. The teachers were both excited, looking forward to the year ahead when they would have the opportunity to mold such potential.

As the year progressed these two classes excelled in the standardized testing, highest in the state; their students won state competitions in several areas. At the end of the school year, the principal met with the two teachers and confessed that the students in their class had been chosen randomly and were not necessarily gifted. The teachers assumed with a glow of pride that they must have been specially chosen for their teaching excellence. The principal confided, once again, that their names had been randomly chosen, picked from a hat filled with all the teachers' names.

So, what are your expectations about your body?

Here's the challenge. Each day, for the next 30 days, notice what your body is doing, listen to it, appreciate each aspect of its complex dynamic process. Journal about it. Maybe even verbalize some positive gratitude. And see if you feel a positive difference.

• • •

Take a moment to write down your answers to these questions:

How connected do you feel to your own body?

_____

_____

_____

_____

Do you treat yourself as well as you treat your best friend? If not, why not?

_____

_____

_____

_____

How can you care for yourself better?

_____

_____

_____

_____

7

The Diagnosis...Not the Whole Story

You touch peoples' hearts in the most profound ways.

You are sitting in the hospital bed, recuperating from pneumonia, finally starting to feel a little better after several days of antibiotics, steroids, and nebulizer treatments. You are looking forward to resuming your life, returning to work, and you vow that you won't touch another cigarette ever again. What did the doctor say to you in the hospital room that day?

"Your tests show that you have COPD/bronchiectasis/pulmonary fibrosis..." But what does that mean? You are filled with thoughts... 'Am I ever going to feel like myself again? Am I simply going to get progressively worse and worse?' Suddenly you are accosted by a million fearful destinies. All your hopes and plans change. The world looks and feels different. And maybe you feel that it is your own fault, a victim of your own foolhardiness.

You check Google. 'COPD is defined as a long-term progressive deterioration of respiratory function characterized by increased difficulty breathing, fatigue, increased mucous production and cough........'. Yes, yes, you know about all that. But no cure? You feel robbed of your life, your potential. How will the bills be paid? You feel you can't do anything about it. The simplest task becomes a strenuous chore and you begin to wonder, "Why try?"

That hospital stay, necessary to help your recovery, added a few extra complications when you weren't looking. Bedrest carries with it a lot of extra problems in your body. It messes up your muscles and bones, your heart and circulatory system, your digestive system and your psyche.

As we age, the speed at which we lose muscle tissue, after just a few days in bed increases dramatically. It is typical that after a week in a hospital bed, your muscle mass has decreased 10 to 15%. So, despite overcoming the lung infection, you probably feel much more tired. It's not so much your lung problem, but lying in bed that makes you feel so drained. Further, the shrinking of your muscles includes your chest muscles; you know, those muscles that are supposed to expand and contract when you breathe? This can make you feel like you have to work harder to inhale. Your joints have stiffened.

You have over 600 muscles in your body. If you don't use them, you lose them. When I worked as a student in the nursing home, I cared for patients who were curled up in fetal positions and could not be uncurled. Their muscles had shortened and shrunk to the point that they were unusable. Hands were clenched, backs hunched, knees drawn up. This doesn't occur anymore as physical therapists and nurses exercise patients daily, stretching and lifting to prevent those contractures from occurring.

Rebuilding your muscles takes a little longer than it did to lose them but starting slow and small, little by little, you can regain your strength and your stamina. Having a progressive plan for walking, stretching, and lifting will get you feeling so much better. Talk to your doctor about an exercise plan and ask about pulmonary rehab.

Lying in a hospital bed can also stop your digestive system from functioning normally, which can also make you feel weak and out of sorts. Lack of movement and medications are big culprits. Confucius, an ancient Chinese sage, once remarked that Constipation is the mother of disease. Regaining your daily cycle will help every other part of your body to function better.

After just a week in bed, your blood may be thicker, and your ability to carry oxygen is decreased. The muscles of your heart get weak so your heartbeat speeds up because it doesn't work as efficiently, impacting your stamina. Once you are back up and active again, your cardiovascular system will return to normal.

Lying in a hospital bed, your mind churns, going over and over the words spoken by your doctor, again and again and again; your brain can't shut off and the more you try to avoid your thoughts, the more they weigh you down, like a massive stone on your shoulders. You feel exhausted before you even begin to move your body.

So, is it your lung disease that is causing you to feel so bad? Which part of your body is it?

• • •

Take a moment to write down your answers to these questions:

What do you think is draining your energy right now?

_____

_____

_____

_____

What action can you do to improve your energy level?

_____

_____

_____

_____

When can you start that action towards improved energy?

_____

_____

_____

_____

How can you schedule it into your day?

_____

_____

_____

_____

8

Joe: Leading the Team

We want to be better... You show us we can.

J oe arrived for his first day of rehab, dressed in his gym shorts and T-shirt. It felt good just to be wearing his work-out clothes again after so long; it made him feel young again, energized, hopeful. But he was also nervous. He wasn't at all sure that he could do much of anything in there. The machines were lined up in rows across the gym and the weights, pretty big weights were stacked in the back corner. "No way," he thought. Joe decided he would just stay relaxed and follow directions, not that he had any expectations. He wondered if Sandy had ever just given up on a patient, if maybe she had gently explained, 'We made a mistake. We don't think this is for you.' Joe's thoughts were grinding his stamina into pieces by the time he crossed the gym. "Would she say that to him? Well, he would just give it his best shot."

Sandy was there waiting for him. "Hi Joe! It's great to see you! Come on in. Let's switch over your oxygen and get you out of that wheelchair onto the chair. You look good." She said. Others, some with oxygen, some without oxygen, were sitting having their blood pressure done and looking at their paperwork. "Hey everyone, this is Joe, first time here." Introductions were made. Jack gave him a welcoming smile and a pat on the back. "Sandy will take good care of you, she's great, but watch out for Mary over there, she's a sergeant," he laughed. Mary, the nurse at the desk, smiled and said, "Oh Jack, you are so full of beans! Welcome, Joe." Betty, David, and Bob said their hellos and sauntered off to the back of the gym to start their stretches. 'Here Comes the Sun' by the Beatles was playing in the background. Sandy switched over Joe's canula to the tank and turned the knob to two liters. She took Joe's blood pressure and his oximetry readings. "Perfect, 134/82, 94%." She knew Joe was nervous and was not surprised to see that the blood pressure was a little high. "Let's get started." They began walking to the back of the gym. "Looks like you've been doing your homework, I can tell by just watching you walk. You look stronger, already." Joe smiled, feeling more at ease than when he first walked in.

Sandy coached him on how to do the stretches posted on the far wall. He was stiff and his muscles were pretty weak, but he rested in between stretches, while Sandy explained breathing techniques, including the golden rule: PLB. Pursed Lip Breathing: 'Smell the roses, blow out the candles'. She talked about how to stretch without overstressing his joints. "Remember, Joe, the tortoise won the race, not the hare. Be smart, go slow, stay focused, and breathe." He was surprised at how difficult a sit-stand exercise was. When she grabbed a cushion so he didn't have to sit so low, it seemed to help some. His homework assignment grew to include stretches as well as his walking.

Getting on the treadmill was a little intimidating. Sandy kept track of his oximetry and stayed with him during the two minutes he walked. It felt good to be in the gym, on a treadmill, working out with the group. He was embarrassed at how slow she set the pace but, he figured, he'd rather take it slow and easy at first. After two minutes, though, he knew it was more challenging than he had expected.

He enjoyed the occasional banter back and forth with the other clients. Jack seemed to get everyone going. "Funny guy," he thought. He enjoyed the nu-step the most and felt like he got a good workout of most of his major muscles, arms and legs, on that one. He was thrilled that he was able to work out on that for three minutes. The bike was tough, not his favorite. A minute on that wiped him out. "Take it easy. Go slow." She kept saying. "I guess this is not exactly like the gym back home where everyone tries to outdo each other. This seems to be mostly just getting those muscles moving again. Makes sense." He thought. After each exercise he had to stop, rest, breathe. Sandy explained to him how to indicate the levels of fatigue and shortness of breath and where to note it on his program sheet. "These numbers help us both recognize your present limits and your future potential," said Sandy, smiling. She had confidence in him, he could feel it, and he didn't want to let her down. He knew he wouldn't let her down.

A few minutes before the end of the session, Sandy gave Joe a kazoo. Rick, the respiratory therapist, led the entire group in some interesting breathing exercises that gave his lungs a good work out. Then, Rick picked up his guitar. Everyone started playing along on the kazoo with the song, "Take it Easy" by the Eagles. "Not quite ready for Carnegie Hall," someone laughed, when the song ended. He did feel like his breathing was a little easier after playing a couple of songs on the kazoo. His oxygen was up to 97%. "That's good," he thought. Rick encouraged him to do some breathing exercises at home and even play the kazoo once in a while. One of the guys mentioned that he was now the official kazoo player at every birthday party.

Rick talked about breathing exercises that could calm him down when he was anxious. He explained the importance of good posture for breathing and had them demonstrate by playing a song on the kazoo slumped in the chair and then sitting up straight. He could feel the difference! And of course, Rick reminded everyone to purse lip breathe when they were using energy to prevent that shortness of breath.

After almost an hour Joe was spent. But it was a good spent, like he had just had a workout and it felt good. "Great job, today, Joe!" Sandy yelled as he walked out of the gym, "See you Thursday!" Joe turned his head and nodded, a smile creeping up the corners of his mouth.

Ellie was waiting for him in the waiting room, eager to hear about the session. "How'd it go?" "Not bad, I guess." He grumbled. He was tired. Ellie noticed some color in his cheeks and she rolled her eyes, pulling up his wheelchair. She knew this was a good idea; he just wasn't going to admit it yet. Joe settled back in the wheelchair, remembering to sit up straight instead of slouching, like he usually did.

Take a moment to write down your answers to these questions:

What are the first three steps that you can take to get you closer to that vision of yourself you created?

_____

_____

_____

What resources can you use to help you get to that vision?

_____

_____

_____

How committed are you to reaching your goals?

_____

_____

_____

How will you plan your progress?

_____

_____

_____

9

Leading Your Team

Each person you touch feels at home, feels appreciated, feels understood.

Recognizing yourself as the leader of a team of healers is essential. This team of healers includes your pulmonologist, pharmacist, rehab nurse, respiratory therapist, exercise physiologist, support group, and most importantly, your family members. A strong team leader has confidence in the team, has high expectations, and is a clear communicator.

All the team members work under you and for you. You are the team leader. You need to be in charge of you.

Your Doctor:

Have a doctor that you are comfortable with, a doctor who listens and who is available when you need them. It's well and good to have a doctor tell you what to do, what to take, and give a professional opinion but it's not enough. You need this doctor to believe in your potential to improve. You are not a statistic or a test result. Statistics are meant to be indicators; they do not reflect the whole picture, the whole you.

The way you feel and the questions you have are really important to share with your pulmonologist. Yes, numbers can be meaningful, but how you feel and what you think is just, if not more, important.

Doctors are often required by corporate administrators to schedule appointments back to back every 20 minutes throughout the day. That gives you very little time. Your time needs to be used efficiently and effectively, by you. This age of technology means that the doctor walks in the room and promptly focuses his eyes and fingers on the computer as he talks with you. Observation is key in determining your condition. Does the physician look at you? If a physician is not open to your feelings, thoughts, or questions, you may want to consider seeing someone else. And if you cannot get in to see your doctor when you need him or her the most, you are not getting your needs met and you may want to consider looking for another option.

When you have appointments with your doctor, I suggest that you always, yes, *always* bring a notebook with specific updates on your condition. If you don't share this information, your doctor won't know. Also, bring, on paper, a list of questions you want to address. Don't leave until you jot down the answers. How often have we all walked out of our scheduled visit, feeling frustrated by our unanswered questions, unsure of what the doctor had just explained.

It's not unusual to have four or five separate doctors, a pulmonologist, cardiologist, endocrinologist, primary care physician, and more. Unfortunately, these doctors do not talk with one another regarding your case and may prescribe treatments or meds that may interfere or interact with others that you are taking. You will have to step up and take responsibility for coordination. Communicate and share with each doctor your medications, treatments, and conditions each time you visit. Always review your full list of medications each time you visit each of your doctors. If you are prescribed a new medication, ask why, what to expect, and if there might be side effects.

Doctors do tend to love numbers, and can be easily impressed if you share trends in blood pressure, oximetry (captured by that little finger device you can get at most drug stores), heart rate, and weight. Informing the physician about how frequently you use your inhaler, how you are managing daily activities, and how you are progressing towards your goals allows him or her to understand a more holistic picture of your health. Tracking, monitoring, and sharing that information presents you as an educated consumer who takes responsibility for your own health.

Your job does not stop there:

It is not the doctor's job to make you well. You need to make you well by taking medications as prescribed and knowing why you are taking them. Following up with the doctor to share effects of the newly prescribed medicine is a big help. Is it working for you or not? Your doctor can't do a good job if s/he thinks you are taking a medication but you had stopped it after a couple of weeks because it didn't agree with you. You need to notify the prescribing doctor if you have any serious side effects or if you find a particular medication to be ineffective.

Jimmy would consult with more than one doctor at times to clarify a concern or a treatment option. He would bring each issue up with his pulmonologist once again, after consulting with the other doctors, the rehab staff, and other patients. His pulmonologist respected his research. He would usually comply with Jim's decision or give clearly stated reasons when he thought the proposed option would not be the best choice. His doctor recognized that Jim was conscientious, he did his homework. He knew Jim was reliable so he gave Jim a prescription for an antibiotic and a steroid. "Take it when you need to and just let me know when you do." His doctor understood that exacerbations happen suddenly sometimes, and usually on a weekend when it is hard for patients to access their doctors and/or new prescriptions.

Researching lung health strategies is as easy as a Google search, and can help you start to fill your tool box of strategies and actions that will improve your health and outlook. Join pulmonary disease chat rooms and learn what others are doing for recovery. Be aware that misinformation and negative chats can mislead you though, so validate any information obtained with your doctor, nurse, pharmacist, or other provider before trying something new. Find your closest pulmonary rehab center and support group. You can learn so much from other clients, and concurrently find yourself among a set of friends who understand your situation.

Louise arrived at pulmonary rehab with significant shortness of breath despite being on five liters of O2. Eventually she needed to increase her O2 even higher when she was exercising until she was obliged to wear a mask in order to increase the percentage of oxygen she could access. Louise, 57 years old, had been divorced for many years, and had no children. She always had a laugh and a smile though. She would arrive breathless and take the few minutes to relax on the bench before starting her exercise routine. She lived alone in an apartment overlooking the park and felt fairly capable of caring for herself. Louise had adopted two parakeets several years ago and she would go on and on about how they chirped and chatted to each other. She loved those parakeets. One day she arrived at rehab with some difficult news. "I saw the doctor on Monday, he said that I need to consider getting a transplant. My lungs are getting worse and he can't increase my O2 any further. My only real worry is that if I do go to the hospital for a transplant, I have no one to take care of my parakeets. I just can't do it."

When the rehab team had their regular team meeting that week, Louise's name came up. The staff members were worried about Louise and noted to Dr. Woods, the rehab's medical director, that she was not doing well. Sandie explained that Louise was most concerned for her parakeets; they were her whole family. Dr. Woods asked if she had been tested for psittacosis, which can exhibit symptoms similar to fibrosis. "Psittacosis is a lung infection caused by bacteria found in our feathered friends. If she has been inhaling this bacterium, she may be experiencing some serious chronic pulmonary inflammation. Let's check with Louise's doctor to find out if they have considered that possibility." Sandy followed up with Louise's doctor to see if this had been checked.

We didn't see Louise for a while, and we worried that she had deteriorated further. She stopped in a month later, her oxygen was down to two liters and her breathing looked much improved. She announced that her breathing was getting better and better; her need for oxygen was lessening, and she felt stronger every day. "You look so much better, Louise. What happened?" "Well, I had to give away my parakeets as they were the reason my lungs were so bad. I found a good home for them so they will be fine." We nodded. "My lungs are much better now and according to the doctor I should return to normal in another few months." Louise had that bounce she always had, but now it was a lot easier for her. She was happy about being healthy once again though she missed her birds. "No more birds for me. I miss them so much, but I know they will be fine. I've been thinking of maybe getting a puppy."

Your Pharmacist:

Compared to your physician who studied all aspects of every disease process, your pharmacist studied, primarily medication, for eight years. Your pharmacist is a valuable resource on how medicine works and how it affects your body.

You should be on a first name basis with your pharmacist. It's important to have one who is aware of every medication you are taking, including the supplements, and any that you buy over the counter. Some medications can have a different effect when combined with certain other medications and some of the effects can be hazardous. Share your concerns. Ask for opinions. If you are having some uncomfortable side effects from a medication, ask the pharmacist for some suggestions or alternative options.

Rehab Professionals: RNs, Exercise Physiologists, and Respiratory Therapists:

In pulmonary rehab, you will work with an RN (registered nurse), an exercise physiologist, and a respiratory therapist. Each is there to prescribe suitable exercises that may include stretches, weights, and aerobic machines. This team of providers will monitor your oxygen levels and your levels of shortness of breath during your exercise. They will also measure your progress and, focus on making you stronger, healthier, and happier. They will give you strategies on improving your overall wellness, including your physical, psychological, social, and emotional wellness. They keep on top of the latest trends in research, introducing you to strategies for easier breathing and better health. These rehab team members will also prescribe respiratory muscle exercises and maybe offer different research-based strategies including tai chi, kazoo, reiki, and/or mindfulness. They are there to monitor your safety and your overall health.

The rehab team is there for clients who need a second opinion on symptoms. Clients can be reassured that the team is supportive and open to them. They will listen to their lungs, check their blood pressure, assess their blood sugar and oxygen levels and assess their clinical status. "Yes, Tom, let's hold off on exercising today. You need to stop in at your doctor's office on the way home. I'll give the office a call and let them know you are coming. You have some crackles in your right lower lobe which is new for you. Hopefully, you have caught it early enough. The doctor may want to take an X-ray and prescribe some antibiotics and maybe prednisone."

Art keeps up with what's happening in the pulmonary treatment trends; he reads the magazines and checks online publications and news sites. He asked his treatment team about marijuana, having researched some information regarding its use with lung disease. "Looks promising…" he said, his eyes searching for some confirmation. Sandy shakes her head. "Too early to tell. Not enough research yet, but it's possible, that this might prove to be helpful. It's worth keeping up on the research." They have discussed supplements and herbs, aromatherapy, acupuncture, and salt chambers, stem cell treatments, and transplants. Art is perpetually discovering new treatments and possible remedies and he keeps his team members on their toes reviewing the studies. This proactive approach serves Art, his treatment team, and all the clients at his rehab center. It also represents the optimistic and engaged attitude that can only hasten improvement!

There are treatments and strategies being discovered every day. It's up to you and your team to keep abreast of the latest trends and treatments. COPD Foundation, American Lung Association, Breathe Strong, and the Pulmonary Paper are great places to start your online investigation.

Support Group:

Support groups are grassroots resources for learning information, sharing ideas and for connecting. In a support group, you suddenly find that you are among friends and you are no longer facing your challenges alone. They can help you find the best oxygen concentrator; they might know where you can get a deal on home air purifiers, or ways to manage on those humid days. The other group members have to handle the same problems you are. If you are having a tough time with some of your daily routines, share that. You'll likely get several ideas on how to make it a lot easier.

Barry complained that his oxygen tubing at home was so long it would kink up. "I use a swivel connector between my extension and the cannula so it doesn't kink up anymore." Replied a member in the group. "It really makes big difference for me. I get it at the medical supply store down on Ash Street." "I stretch out the tubing on top of my car on a warm sunny afternoon and it relaxes all the kinks." Said another.

Clara got very short of breath in the morning with her shower. It would take all her effort and when she was finished, she would be exhausted for the rest of the day. "Are you wearing your oxygen in the shower? You should be." "Don't put your oxygen concentrator in the shower, just use your canula with a long extension." "The steam can be tough. Try lowering the temperature of the water a bit and open the window and door; turn on the fan if you have one." "And sit down. It's much easier to wash your hair by lowering your head." "And if you have one of the nice big Sheraton towel robes from Big Lots, you can wrap that around you and let the robe dry you off while you are sitting." Everyone in the group seemed to have a helpful solution.

Clara came in two weeks later and raved about how much easier showering was since she used a few of those idea. "That fluffy white robe really works wonders. I actually still have some energy left after my shower!"

Family:

Your family members and/or friends are vital members of your team. They are the ones who remind you of the questions to ask the team, they remind you to do your exercise homework, and they provide you with the support and encouragement you sometimes need. And on those days that aren't your best, they will run down to the store and grab those items that were on your shopping list, help with your medication management, and notice when you may need to make an appointment to see the doctor. One of the signs of low oxygen is confusion and sleepiness. Your wife, or a good friend may notice that your oxygen tubing is kinked or has become disconnected. Don't forget to show appreciation for their help. And on those good days, remember to help them out in return.

Be sure to tell family and friends about your lung disease. It helps them to understand and support you when you need it, and we all need it at times.

· · ·

Take a moment to write down your answers to these questions:

Who is on your support team?

_____

_____

_____

Who else would be helpful to have on your team?

_____

_____

_____

How can you utilize your team more effectively?

_____

_____

_____

What change or action can you take to get the most benefit?

_____

_____

_____

10

Joe: A Rediscovery

You helped me see what really matters.

66 What's most important for you, Joe?" "My family, I guess, getting my life back and supporting my family."

"How would you like to see yourself a year from now, Joe?"

"Well, I'd like to be happy, be able to do more things."

"Like what?"

"Like go back to work, play golf with the guys, ...and help out a little at home, you know... fix that broken light in the hall, and do some yardwork, you know."

Joe started to think about what really was most important to him. "...Ellie," he thought. Ellie was most important to him, and not feeling like an anchor around her neck. "I just really want Ellie to be happy again," he thought. Joe looked out the window at the trees lining the sidewalk across the street and the mountains in the distance. He looked back at Sandy and sighed. "You know, I'd just really like to take a walk with my wife, in the morning in the park, across the street from our house." Joe smiled and looked down, lost in thought.

"And how are you feeling when you are doing that, Joe?"

"Great. I feel great. It's a sunny day. She's holding my hand and she looks at me the way she used to, not with pity."

"How do you look?" Joe looks up.

"I'm smiling."

• • •

There is a wise old Chinese proverb that states that hell is a place of starvation, frustration, and anguish. In the center of hell, is a large bowl of rice and each member surrounding this bowl of rice have such very long chopsticks they can't reach their mouth with the rice they have on their chopsticks. They are starving and in anguish.

Heaven is the same scenario, but it is full of joy and sustenance. Once again, there is a large bowl of rice surrounded by a group of people with the same long chopsticks. The difference is simply that, in heaven, they are happy to feed each other.

We need to allow others to help us just as we need to help. It goes both ways.

In getting out of ourselves and our own stories, showing compassion and connection to others, we feel more alive and engaged in life! By helping others and by allowing others to help us, we become an integral part of the dynamic life process. We have purpose.

The oncology surgeon, Dr. Siegel, described a personal story in his book, *Love, Medicine and Miracles*. He became incapacitated with severe back strain unable to move without searing bursts of pain across his back. The hospital called and notified him that his patient who had an enlarged tumor pressing against his vital organs required immediate surgery in order to survive. There was no other surgeon who could do the surgery. So, Dr. Siegel scheduled the operation for first thing in the morning. When morning arrived, he pulled himself out of bed, hobbled his way to his car and drove to the hospital. As he planned to perform surgery, he knew he could not take any medications to ease the pain; he needed to be completely alert and focused. Holding his back, bent and in anguish, Dr. Siegel found his way to the scrub room, where he leaned over the sink and scrubbed up. Still bent over, he opened the door into the surgical suite where he saw his patient draped and ready.

In an instant he became completely focused. Working with his well-tuned staff, he operated for six hours without stopping, completely engrossed in the task. Upon completion, he removed his gown and gloves, smiled, thanked the staff, and walked out the door. As soon as he was out of the surgical suite, he doubled over, bent, and in anguish. He remembered his back. Suddenly, he realized that he had completely forgotten about his back; he hadn't felt any pain at all in the previous six hours.

Jack was 50 years old. He was a pilot, a crop duster, spraying fields with insecticides. Long-term inhalation of the toxic chemicals used in the insecticides over the years had its effects on his lungs. After a severe COPD exacerbation, Jack was not able to return to work. He was tired most of the time and his breathing was up and down. Good some days, not so good on other days. All he knew was flying, and he was eager to return to work, but his wife and his doctor absolutely refused to allow him to get even close to that work again. The fumes from those chemicals had done such damage to his lungs. He was young though and he still had lots of energy; well, he did but his body didn't. He began to feel useless and dependent, and slowly he began to do less and less at home. He was at a pretty low point when his friend, Mike, asked him if he might be able to help out down at the local community dining room for the homeless.

That's where Sandy met Jack, 5 years later, pouring out juice and milk to the guests that arrived for the meal. She noticed how the guests all seemed to know him. They would stand around the juice table exchanging jokes with Jack. She asked Jack about his lungs, one day, seeing the oxygen canister by his side. Sandy suggested that he might enjoy attending rehab. Jack took to Rehab like a fish. He's been a regular now for the past several years and everyone knows him by name. He is the first one to welcome the newbies, making them feel comfortable.

Jack isn't despondent anymore. He's too busy to think about himself. Besides his work with the homeless and going to rehab, he has a huge email group whose members look forward to his daily jokes and interesting facts.

By sharing and helping others we forget about our own troubles.

Pulmonary rehab is a community of people dealing with common issues: shortness of breath, weakness, fatigue, mucous, medicines, oxygen tanks and concentrators. It is an ever-growing family who work together toward common goals: to breathe easier and to live fully engaged in the world. They help each other. Although I am a nurse and educator, the best teachers are the clients themselves. They understand, they help, and they share with each other.

• • •

Take a moment to write down your answers to these questions:

What do you value the most in life?

_____

_____

_____

_____

How do your goals and vision compare to your most valued?

_____

_____

_____

_____

If you needed someone who would you call? Who could you help out today?

_____

_____

_____

_____

11

So, What is Chronic Lung Disease? Really.

*You have supported me, taught me, shared with
me, laughed with me and cried with me.*

There are about 37 million people in the US alone who carry the diagnosis of Chronic Lung Disease. It is the third most-common medical diagnosis. So why don't we see or hear more about it than we do?

Chronic Lung disease is treatable. It's not a terminal illness. It can be uncomfortable and require extra attention, but many clients I've known, in stage three, which is sometimes referred to as 'end stage' lung disease, are still working and enjoying life. Whatever stage you are in, the way you feel and the state of your lungs is very unique to you. No two are the same. Some of my clients with stage one and two, mild to moderate lung disease, are much more debilitated, short of breath and fatigued. Is it the lungs or is it the attitude? Many 'end stage' patients have been attending pulmonary rehab for several years.

The better we care for ourselves, our overall health, the more likely we are to stay healthy.

COPD is an overall term describing a partial blockage in the process of breathing. The airway is not clear and open because of swelling, muscle tightness, or excess mucous. Emphysema is frequently an associated part of COPD. Emphysema is injury to the balloon-like structures throughout your lungs, called alveoli. With Emphysema, there is injury to these structures, where the exchange of oxygen and carbon dioxide occurs. In the past, we associated this with 'smokers' lung'. That's because smoking is the number one cause of COPD. But at least 20 percent of people with COPD never smoked.

If you do smoke, quitting is your best bet on slowing the progress of the disease and it will improve your symptoms. Find the way that works best for you. Get support. Chantix has been a useful tool for many ex-smokers. Ask your team for ideas. There are a variety of proven strategies.

Lil was a 34-year-old who never smoked, but suffered from the fatigue and shortness of breath of severe lung disease due to her cancer treatments. She was a tech working in the IT department at the hospital when she was diagnosed. Lil was treated successfully with chemo and was eager to return to work, but a recent lung infection identified irreversible lung damage. Lil's weight was down to 90 pounds and her stamina was waning. Her doctor advised a transplant. But to be strong enough for a transplant, she needed to regain some weight on her 64-inch gaunt frame, rebuild her strength and regain her stamina. It was an effort for her to push herself up from the wheelchair to a standing position. Walking for thirty seconds drained her. But she was determined. Unless she regained some strength, she would not be a healthy enough candidate for the surgery. Lil worked hard, both at rehab and at home, increasing her walking to almost three minutes and improving her weight. It was slow going and we were worried about her. Mary, the nurse, had faith in her. "Lil is too stubborn to give up. She's going to make it, I just know."

Finally, Lil got the call. Her bag had been packed for several weeks. Because of her frail condition, she had risen up the list to priority status. A week later, she called the rehab team from her hospital room. "Everything went great. I'm already up and walking. Can't seem to stop doing my pursed lip breathing even though it's so easy now to breathe." She laughed. You could hear the joy in her voice. There were lots of happy tears that day in rehab.

When you breathe, the air enters your nose or mouth and flows down the bronchial passage, where it branches off to the right and left until it reaches the alveoli. You have three lobes or sections of lung in your right chest, and two lobes or sections near your heart, in your left. Alveoli are arranged in clusters of sacs, like clusters of grapes. There are millions of these alveolar sacs in your lungs. Each alveolus is like a balloon. When you inhale, the air flows through your bronchial tree and expands these alveoli like balloons. Blood vessels surround these sacs and as the alveoli fill up with air, the oxygen seeps over into the bloodstream to be carried to the rest of the body while carbon dioxide seeps into the alveoli to be expelled with exhalation. As you exhale, the balloons of the alveoli constrict, just like a balloon.

COPD is an obstruction of that process and usually impacts the bronchial tube or airway itself as well as the alveoli. It's a term that encompasses a variety of lung situations, each of which in some way, obstructs that flow.

Asthma is an inflammation and a tightening of the bronchial tubes usually brought on by a trigger; exercise, cold, stress, overexertion, or illness can bring on an attack.

Cystic Fibrosis is an overproduction of mucous in the airways, causing blockage.

Bronchiectasis, can be considered a type of cystic fibrosis involving once again, an overproduction of mucous in your airway preventing easy breathing.

Chronic bronchitis and bronchiolitis involve inflammation of the bronchial tube causing a narrowing of the airway. Each type obstructs the process of accessing air through your airway,

COPD very often includes damage to the alveoli preventing some of those balloon-like structures from transferring the oxygen into the blood vessels. Some of your air sacs lose their elasticity, like a balloon that has been blown up too long. When you release the opening to the balloon, the air simply sits inside and is not interested in being expelled.

The problem with COPD is not as much difficulty breathing in, but difficulty breathing out. You need to expel that dead air in your alveoli before you can access fresh air back into them. This can be alleviated with pursed lip breathing. When you pursed lip breathe you are pushing the air out of your lungs, squeezing those balloons so that with your next breath, you can take in more air deeper into your alveoli.

Pulmonary fibrosis is a scarring that occurs in your lung tissue. Some of the alveoli have developed a thickened membrane preventing oxygen from seeping through to the blood vessels. Using oxygen while exercising, with pursed lip breathing, will help enhance the efficiency of your lungs.

Restrictive lung disease occurs when the lungs are unable to expand and fill completely. It's not unusual to have some of both, restrictive and obstructive. Curvature of the spine, paralyzed diaphragm or an inability of the chest wall to expand would prevent the lungs from inhaling to full capacity. Again, remember, our lungs are huge. How many of us breathe to our full capacity and how frequently?

Gerry was anxious about his decreased lung capacity, having recently undergone a pneumonectomy for lung cancer. Although his cancer was treated, he was afraid to push himself in fear that he would lose his breath. "You have a lung, three whole lobes, Gerry. That's plenty. God gave us way more lung power than we ever use. That lung extends below your rib cage. It's pretty big. You'll do fine. And here in rehab, you will get that lung working even more efficiently." Rick, the respiratory therapist explained. "You aren't a deep-sea diver, though are you? You might consider another sport."

Kurt is a husband and father of three young children. He works in maintenance in the local school district. The job requires lifting and carrying, climbing ladders and stairways. Initially he was afraid to tell his boss about his oxygen requirement and avoided using his oxygen at work. He knew that his oxygen saturation was critically low, in the 60s at times with some of the strenuous work that he was doing, but he was so afraid that he would lose his job, he avoided the issue. He had to work; his family needed him. He began attending pulmonary rehab before work in the morning and he shared his fear of his family's economic insecurity due to his lung disease. His pulmonologist encouraged him to go for a transplant, but he didn't feel ready for that.

Kurt never missed a day of work, and was understandably scared that his job may not be safe if his lung disease became public, or he had to take time off for a transplant. However, no one can legally lose his job due to their need for oxygen. For his health he must use oxygen. The rehab team encouraged him to sit down and explain to his boss that his performance at work, which was already more than satisfactory according to his annual evaluations, would improve even more. Further, his ability to continue working would be much more sustainable and he would continue to be able to care for his family.

Kurt finally sat down and explained his health situation to his boss. She was more than accepting of Kurt wearing his oxygen. She even said that she would follow up with him regularly to make sure he was using it at work. Kurt felt touched by his boss's concern over his health and well-being, and he was thrilled that he would now be able to avoid transplant surgery a little longer.

When we are responsible for someone or something, we tend to push ourselves a little harder. Those mornings that getting out of bed seems like an enormous task, the thought of something, or someone else can turn it into a difficult, but do-able obstacle. There is no choice but to get up and go to work. People are depending on us! In rehab, your team is depending on you to show up. And when you do, despite the effort it took, you feel great about making it.

Pulmonary disease is usually diagnosed through pulmonary function tests. During these tests, your nose is clamped and you breathe forcefully through a tube that measures the volume, the force, the speed, and the duration of your breath. Results can vary depending on many factors, including how you are breathing that particular day, how stressed you are, and how well you slept the night before. The test will be repeated until the therapist perceives that you have accurately carried out the task. There are no 100% scores. Normal ranges are between 70 or 80. So when you got your results of 50, did you understand that the normal is 70%?

Oximetry measures the percentage of oxygenated hemoglobin in your bloodstream. It's a simple finger device that you can buy for as little as $30.00. You can also download an app that can measure your oxygen by directing the laser light onto your finger. This is an important self-diagnostic tool with which you can quickly and easily check your oxygen level. Your oxygen level usually should stay above 88% or whatever number your physician suggested. Some people cope with levels lower than normal and seem to adapt to it, going about their daily tasks. Some people can feel short of breath when their oxygen numbers are within normal, and some people have low oxygen levels without shortness of breath. The experience of lung disease is unique to each person.

CT scans and X-rays may or may not give an indication of where in your lungs an injury is located.

A simple blood test can determine if there is a genetic anomaly resulting in Alpha1 Antitrypsin. This diagnosis can be treated with ongoing medication that will maintain your lung capacity and prevent progression of lung damage. The key factor is to identify it before it gets too far along.

COPD is a diagnosis, a label. You are not the label. You simply have a respiratory issue. You need to differentiate between you and the label. You are not a COPD patient, or a pulmonary fibrosis patient. You are someone who has a lung issue that, with the appropriate medications and treatments is being controlled. With flexibility and common sense, you continue on with life.

You have two lungs with a total of 5 lobes, and 600 million alveoli. When the doctor declares that you have only 50% of your lung capacity, be happy. God gave you much more lung power than you ever normally use. How often do we ever actually use much of our lung capacity? Unless you are a sprinter or a deep-sea diver, you might not miss a few thousand alveoli.

• • •

Take a moment to write down your answers to these questions:

What is your diagnosis and what symptoms do you have?

_____

_____

_____

_____

What have you done so far to improve your lung health?

_____

_____

_____

_____

What action can you take that might help you breathe better and feel stronger?

_____

_____

_____

_____

12

Minding your Mind

You believe in me.

A physician was doing rounds one day in the hospital checking in on his patients, reviewing the results of their tests, scans and bloodwork. He was in a hurry that day, as he had a busy schedule and was already running behind. He was a good physician, pragmatic and up front with his patients, well respected, and hard working. As he reviewed the scans, he found the report on the growing metastatic cancer. He enters the patient's room, sits down with him and his wife and says, "I have some difficult news for you. According to your tests, you have metastatic cancer, too advanced for any surgical intervention and it appears that you don't have long to live. I'm sorry." The physician left and moved on to his next task. It was a while later when he suddenly learned that he had spoken to the wrong patient. This scan belonged to the patient across the hall. The physician quickly returned to report his error to the patient, but the damage was done. Unfortunately, the patient who had been hospitalized for a simple hernia repair went home, became sicker and sicker and finally died within three months.

Our minds absorb the words of a physician as the word of God, as if the entire control of our health lies in his/her unlimited wisdom. Often times we fail to recognize the role that we ourselves play in our healing. Remember the intuitive intelligence of one single cell in our body. We often dismiss our own amazing capacity to heal. Belief can limit or enhance our potential to heal ourselves.

Chuck was steadily progressing in his rehab program. He was walking the track in the gym, feeling great about his progress. Chuck would always have a witty remark to loosen up the group and get them chuckling as they did their stretches. He was gaining confidence and he would encourage the new participants who sometimes struggled. One day, Chuck arrived at rehab and found that he just didn't have the stamina to complete his laps as usual. He was quieter than usual, and we couldn't get any witty retorts from him. We knew something was going on. Sandy sat down next to him, concerned. "Tough day today, Chuck? Did you sleep okay? Your lungs sound good. How's your breathing?" "I saw my doctor yesterday," Chuck said. "He told me not to buy any green bananas." Chuck shakes his head and chuckles. "What do you mean?" Sandy had a quizzical look. "I'm not going to live long enough to see them ripen, I guess." "Chuck, you are doing amazing, you have come so far and done so well, you are up to 10 minutes on the track and looking great! That doesn't make any sense!"

Chuck went home without completing the class and he did not return. Sandy called several times but always got the answering machine. Chuck didn't return any of the calls.

Focus on how you feel, not on the results of a test. Who knows if it might have been an off day for you, or test results could have been impacted by a distracting thought, a sleepless night, or maybe some excess phlegm. Numbers and test results change. It doesn't necessarily mean that you have changed. "My lung function tests got better." Betty said. "I feel the same. Maybe it's the exercise."

Find a doctor who believes in you, not the disease. Yes, you have something that needs to be addressed. There are lots of ways to handle this issue. You, like all of us, need a supportive team to help you. A physician who believes in your ability to be well and stay well, can improve your wellness capacity immensely.

Deborah would create an excuse to see Dr. Woods almost weekly. Deborah had severe COPD and attended pulmonary rehab conscientiously. She was 72, a smoker for most of her life, and knew that she had not always taken the best care of her health. She was high strung and would tend to try to do too much too fast until she exhausted herself. She was full of life though, always ready to organize the next luncheon or help find the next speaker at the support group meeting. Deborah would feel some congestion, start using her inhaler more, or just feel more run down and she would make an appointment. Deb always felt better when she left Dr. Wood's office. He would spend time listening to her stories, laughing with her jokes and patiently reassuring her. "You are doing fine, stop worrying, Deborah. Keep up the good work…. And check in with me anytime, it's always great to see you!" Dr. Woods cared about Deborah, supported her, and was always there for her. It was his belief in her that kept Deborah so healthy. When exacerbations strike, they can strike fast, and Deborah did end up in the hospital several times. But she pulled herself up each time, starting back up slowly, until she resumed her activity level. She knew the drill, had the tools, and had the support to do it.

The placebo effect is a well-documented occurrence in which a non-drug can be as effective as a drug, depending on the belief of the patient. Thirty percent of control groups, the groups who are given a non-drug in pharmaceutical studies, improve and the reason is because the patients believe that they are taking an actual drug. What exactly is a placebo? A placebo is a substance with no known medical effects, such as sterile water, saline solution, or a sugar pill. A placebo is a fake treatment that in some cases can produce a very real response. The mind is a powerful tool in our capacity to be well.

Use your mind. Every time you take your medication, say to yourself: **This medicine is keeping me healthy and strong. This medicine is keeping me breathing easily. I breathe so much better and feel so much better when I take this medicine.** See yourself in your mind's eye, breathing easy, feeling great.

'... Two and a half to three and a half years to live...' The words rippled across Brent's monitor screen again and again. That is what he absorbed. Okay. That's it then. So, being realistic, he immediately completed all important end of life plans and prepared himself and his family for his demise.

Brent was referred to Dr. Woods, the pulmonologist, by his primary care physician. His primary care physician had shared with Brent that he appeared to have some pulmonary fibrosis and COPD. Brent was an engineer and of course the first task was to investigate these terms.

His wife, Barb, who accompanied Brent at this appointment, was still in shock at Brent's findings on the internet. "He looks so good, Dr. Woods, and he is so strong, I still can't believe that this could happen from a simple respiratory infection." Barb's face was ashen and worn. Brent relayed his doctor's suspicions and his own findings online to Dr. Woods who returned his gaze to the screen behind him to recheck Brent's x-ray. Dr. Woods brought them both over to the x-rays on the wall. "These are your lungs, Brent. See that tiny spot at the tip of your lower lobe there?" he pointed, "that might be a little spot of fibrosis; it could have been there since you were born, who knows ...and I can see a slight thickening along the bronchial tree.....But you look fine to me, Brent. Your clinical picture looks fine. You have a lot of years to live and enjoy without worry. I don't see any fibrosis or any obstructive process that's significant." Brent's and Barb's eyes widened with the news; color rushed into their faces as they took in his words. "Oh!" Brent said, regaining his composure. "Well, you are the pulmonologist, and the best so I'm told. Wow, that's very reassuring. Thank you, Doctor." "Doctor Woods, that is wonderful, wonderful news! Thank you!" Barb laughed with obvious relief as she through her arms around him.

Although we have easy access to information online. It doesn't mean that it is all true. You can find everything and anything online. Beware of any web sites that give you negative reports. The only time that people feel the need to write about a treatment or disease in a chat is often when they have a complaint. The thousands of people without issues, are too busy living life to spend it complaining. If you don't like the diagnosis, get another opinion. And always, always ask your pulmonologist. And if you don't like his opinion, find another pulmonologist to ask. Be sure.

We all have our issues and we all adapt to them in the best way we can. Some of these issues may be evident, like blindness or amputations. Others, like COPD, heart disease, diabetes, or depression are not that evident on the outside. The key to unlocking hidden fears may be to have a clear understanding of what your doctor is telling you and what the possibilities are for being your best. Expect the best, and be grateful.

• • •

Take a moment to write down your answers to these questions:

Which circumstances prevent you from carrying out your action towards your goals?

_____

_____

_____

_____

How can you alter your situation so that you have more influences that help you reach your goals?

_____

_____

_____

_____

How can you minimize those circumstances that hinder you in your progress?

_____

_____

_____

_____

13

Moving Out of Your Comfort Zone

*You see us for who we are and open the way
for us to see that we can achieve.*

The book, *Who Moved My Cheese*, tells the story of two mice that lived in a small mouse hole in the corner of the kitchen. Each morning and evening the two mice would venture out of their mouse hole while everyone was sleeping. On the counter was the round wooden cheese board. The cheese board always had plenty of crumbs and nuggets for the two mice to enjoy. These two mice were content.

One day the two mice ventured onto the counter to find the cheeseboard with the cheese nuggets gone. They sighed forlornly, and returned, hungry, back to their mouse hole. "Tomorrow." They said to each other. The following day, there was still no cheese to be found. Each day for a week, they repeated the trek, finding no cheese. They were getting weaker and hungrier. Finally, one mouse decided that it was time to move on and search for food elsewhere. The other mouse stubbornly refused to consider a change, certain that the cheese would return. The first mouse packed up, said a sad goodbye to his lifelong friend and departed to search for food. As he scurried about exploring options, he found a new home in the house next door. There, he spied a marble cheeseboard with nuggets of cheese along with plenty of cracker crumbs up in the cupboard. He settled in and continued to thrive. The second mouse who had stayed behind, continued to check each day for the cheese but each day he found none. He became weaker and weaker until he finally gave up.

We each have our story, our routine, our views. We are comfortable within our story. It may not be a happy story, but it is ours and it helps us rationalize our choices allowing us to settle into a comfortable, familiar misery. Have we consigned ourselves to this narrow perspective of our potential? It takes energy and courage to change. But in taking this risk, we can edit our story into something better, something meaningful.

Life brings change. And that change is most often unexpected. How do you react to change? Do you get frustrated and angry, or do you get challenged finding new and better ways to adapt and to live? How do you feel about moving on and finding balance? Is it easy? No, but with effort comes huge rewards.

Climbing to the mountain summit, recently, I felt my lungs tighten and my muscles cramp, my legs felt like concrete with each step forward. Suddenly I was over the top and on the descent. The memory of that strain faded fast as I relished the feeling of renewed energy and achievement.

Refuse to be a victim. We all need extra help sometimes and giving someone the opportunity to help is a gift. And you will pay it forward in many ways. Recognize and appreciate who you are, what you have, and what you can do. If you try, despite your fear of failure, you will be better than if you don't try. As previously suggested, tell family and friends about your lung disease. It helps them to understand and support you when you need it and we all need it at times.

Alison was a twenty-year-old nursing student, flying home for her semester break. Exams had been tough and she was ready for some relaxation time at home. Suddenly, she woke to find herself collapsed in the aisle. Cabin attendants were pulling her up in the chair. Alison felt numb. Her breathing was ragged and her whole body felt heavy. A doctor who happened to be on the flight recommended that the airline land at the first available city so she could be cared for.

After two months in the ICU, followed by months of extended care, Alison returned home to her parents'. Doctors decided that she had succumbed to an unknown virus that had left her with muscle weakness and damaging scars on her lungs. There was nothing they could do except help treat her symptoms as best they could. They had no hope she would be functional again and suggested that she accept and move on as best she could.

Alison, frail, wan, with wispy auburn hair, arrived at rehab eager to begin her next phase of recuperation. Though she sat hunched in her wheelchair with her oxygen concentrator attached, there was a distinct spark in her green eyes and a determined look on her face. Despite what doctors and specialists had said, Alison had decided that she was going to regain her independence. And she would.

Though she walked a few steps with a walker, her gait was unsteady. She began her program slowly. Within a few weeks Alison was using the walker more and more and doing up to one lap around the gym on good days. Seeing her step by step progress spurred her on and her confidence grew. Her doctor, impressed with her progress, suggested that a lung transplant might be possible now that she had regained some strength. She would have to gain weight first, and she would have to continue to gain strength in order to survive the surgery.

Alison and her parents met with the dietician to plan out a calorie dense meal schedule. Although she had no appetite, she forced herself to eat. The rehab staff and crew adopted Alison, supporting her through the rigorous testing and the never-easy exercise schedule. The team praised her successes and encouraged her on the tougher days. She was finally up to walking 750 feet and she had gained four pounds when she got the go ahead. She made the transplant list. Because of her age and frailty, her position was very close to the top.

Bags were packed and everyone waited for the news. "Just imagine that phone call in your mind, feel your excitement as you jump in the car and ride to the hospital to receive your new lungs. Imagine breathing easily and feeling great."

Two weeks later, the rehab team received the phone call from the hospital. Ali had received her new set of lungs and with it, a new chance at life. "I feel great!" she said, "The surgery was Wednesday morning and I was out of the intensive care on Friday. I'm already up, walking on my own!" When she stopped in to visit two months later, Alison shared her plans to return to school the following semester. Her boundless determination to resume her life, despite what others said, did not initially include a transplant, but things have a way of working out when you set your eyes on your goal. Alison was an example of success that kept others pushing forward during their tough times. Opportunities will be there if you dare to expect them.

"I was afraid to go out, afraid to be seen tethered to this oxygen albatross. Children stare at me with the oxygen canister on my shoulder like I was a leper. I can't do it."

We all want to fit in. Our self-perception is often unforgiving. We compare ourselves to models and actresses. Whether we are less beautiful or more beautiful, we always sell ourselves short. It's the job of our ever-critical ego to ensure that we come up short. But, isn't it interesting, if we stop and think of some of the most elegant people we have encountered, we may discover that elegance is often unrelated to appearance? It seems that it is more related to a presence, an air of confidence, and a joy in living.

We have the right and the responsibility to engage in our community with or without oxygen tanks.

Liz organized the monthly lunches in local cafes and restaurants. Everyone was welcome. Patients would meet after their rehab to connect and share. It was a friendly group tradition where new and old members found friends. The stigma that so many feel about wearing oxygen in public became a non-issue. It became too common a sight to even notice anymore.

Esther is discouraged when she thinks about the upcoming weekend she and her husband have planned, an evening out at an upscale restaurant with friends. Esther is an elegant woman, impeccable in speech, behavior and appearance. "I get all dressed up to look my best and then I have to put on my oxygen and it simply ruins it." Esther is confessing at the support group meeting.

Happily, someone shows her the latest trend in O2 canula alternatives, a pair of glasses in which the oxygen tubing connects to the temples of the frame behind the ear. Tiny plastic prongs extend from the nose piece of the glasses, diminishing the appearance of the nasal canula to barely noticeable. She is thrilled.

Jerry dyed his long beard green figuring that "If someone is noticing me, it will probably not be because of my oxygen."

Karen, rather than getting embarrassed when she is faced with inquisitive children, appreciates the opportunity to share with them. She explains that because of a problem in her lungs, she needs the extra oxygen from her machine in order to help her breathe more easily. She stresses to them to never smoke and always take care of their lungs because they are precious. It makes her feel good to see the smile and the spark of understanding in their faces. Karen is a

CEO of a nonprofit. She regularly travels, giving lectures to groups of employees and reporting to boards. Her oxygen is her life saver and she treats it like gold. She knows it allows her to continue to do the important work that she does. **Heroes inspire.**

Life can be full of adventures that require little physical energy but can greatly enhance your well-being. Learn to adapt. Move out of your comfort zone.

Which mouse are you? Are you able to adapt and seek out where the cheese moved or are you going to stay put in your same old mind set and wait for things to return to the way they were?

If the story you're living is not forward reaching, close the chapter and open a new one. Do not get stuck in the old negative story....

- ▸ Be your own advocate!!

- ▸ Be adaptable

• • •

Take a moment to write down your answers to these questions:

What might be an action that you could start today to get you closer to doing what you want to do and being who you want to be?

_____

_____

_____

What will you need to carry out this new action?

_____

_____

_____

What have you found (people, places or things) that have helped or that might help you reach your goal?

_____

_____

_____

How can you handle setbacks?

_____

_____

_____

14

The Power of Breath

*You remind us that we are alive in a wonderful
world full of gifts, lessons, and challenges.*

Breathing is something we have, in the past, taken for granted. A natural autonomic function, we gave no thought to it for most of our lives, much like our heartbeat. It functions while we are awake or asleep. It speeds up or slows down depending on what we are doing and feeling. Suddenly, it has become a huge focus in our lives. We are always aware of it, and always fearful of losing our breath.

Your lungs are like balloons that have been blown up too long. Did you ever untie a balloon after it has been inflated for a long time? You open the balloon and the air simply stays inside. The balloon's elasticity has been lost. That's what might be occurring in your lungs. When you inflate your lungs, the air is inhaled but when you exhale, your alveoli, those balloons, simply hold on to that air so that when you try to take in your next breath, there is insufficient space. Getting rid of that dead air has to happen first. You can do that by pursing your lips and blowing out through tight lips, like you were playing the flute. 'Smell the rose; blow out the candle'. You may have seen marathon runners using this technique as it really helps get rid of the dead air and make room for fresh air to enter.

This is especially useful when you are starting to exert yourself. While ascending a flight of stairs you would begin pursed lip breathing first, simply to increase the absorption of oxygen in your system. Then, as you are stepping up to that first stair you are blowing air out. Hesitate as you breathe in through your nose, then, as you are stepping up to the next stair you are blowing out. Take your time and see how you do. Pause when you need to.

Lindsay was traveling home to visit her family back in Massachusetts. Her mom had a two-story house and Lori knew she was going to have to figure out a way to climb those stairs. She started doing a small incline on the treadmill, going really slow, as she did her pursed lip breathing. Lindsay was on two liters of oxygen but when she was exercising, she would increase it up to 4 liters to keep her oxygen levels up. She stuck with it for the two months before her trip. I suggested that maybe she might just ask her mother if she could sleep in the downstairs living room while she was there but Lindsay was too embarrassed. She was the youngest of the three daughters and she wanted to put on her best effort so her 89-year-old mother would not worry about her. Lindsay refused to give up. She returned two weeks later, beaming. She did it. She made sure that she had what she needed when she descended in the morning so she only had to face it once a day but she was ecstatic. "It worked perfectly." she said, "I did my pursed lip breathing and I took my time. It was a lifesaver!"

She shared pictures of her family, smiling and laughing together enjoying the foliage of the Massachusetts autumn. They had been so happy to see her and were pleasantly surprised on how wonderful she looked.

We tend to sit too often, with really poor posture and we breathe shallowly. Simply by improving our posture, by sitting up straight we can improve our capacity to breathe. Pretend for a moment that you are a trumpet player in the band. Slump back in your chair and try to play that trumpet to your favorite song. Hold that note.

Now sit on the edge of your chair with back straight and shoulders back. Try it again? Can you hold that note a little longer?

Simply moving more frequently will show positive results in breathing and in your energy. Stretch out. Take some sighs. Do you have an incentive spirometer? Use it. We know that muscle tightness in our chest can increase the work of breathing. Try exercising your breathing muscles.

Anxiety tightens the chest and decreases your ability to breathe. Focusing on breathing exercises tends to release that tightness, and allow easier breathing.

Have you ever watched a baby breathe? His belly expands and contracts. How do you breathe? Most of us tend to stretch our chest and not our diaphragm. Our diaphragm, the large muscle that acts like a bellows for our lungs becomes lazy.

Both in Tai Chi and Yoga, the breath is central to the practice. Practicing special breathing techniques can increase strength and vitality while stretching and expanding lung capacity. The primary technique involves inhaling deeply, stretching your diaphragm and expanding your belly. As you continue to inhale, your chest fills and finally your shoulders rise, filling your lungs like you were filling a jar, from the bottom of the lungs up to the top. Hold it for a couple of seconds, if you can. Then, release your breath like you are pouring water from a jar, tipping it over, releasing the top, the middle, and finally the bottom of the lungs, completely. Try breathing this way for a few minutes This can really improve oxygenation, as well as decrease your stress and anxiety.

Try taking an extra sip or two of air after your lungs are full. This simply stretches your breathing muscles, exercising them with the theory that by expanding your breathing muscles a little, the job of inspiring becomes a little easier.

When you have relaxed with exhalation, try pushing out a few more drops of air, squeezing the last bit out.

The xi xi hu is a three-part exercise to strengthen the lungs. It is done by taking a belly breath inspiration then a second inspiration and then releasing.

Ujjayi breathing, the buzz breathe, involves inhaling deeply and gently and exhaling closing our throat slightly, creating a soft buzzing sound. This is a stress and anxiety releaser. It may also improve your exhalation.

With any breathing strategy, it's important to stay relaxed; don't strain and don't overdo it. In Tai Chi, the rule is that you only stretch to 70% of your capacity, never pushing yourself too hard. Allow your body the opportunity to be who it is. If you get dizzy, stop. If you are coughing, stop and breathe gently. This is not a competition.

Take time to do some breathing exercises each morning.

Activities that use your breathing muscles can be helpful. As mentioned earlier, we have spent years not using those muscles much, barely breathing and not exercising as much as we should. Muscles get weak, tired and they shorten without use.

Playing kazoo, or any wind instrument and singing is a great way to make wonderful music and stretch those lung muscles. Joining a kazoo group or a singing group is fun and has benefits physically, socially and emotionally. When we incorporated a voluntary kazoo class into the pulmonary rehab program, people started noticing that their breathing became a little more open. They also noticed that their oxygen numbers were better after the kazoo songs.

The Breathing Gym is a series of exercises created by the ASU marching band directors. They started noticing that their musicians were more relaxed allowing more focus when they played and thus more precision. Interestingly, during the summer tour, the band members who had asthma didn't use their inhalers as much as they used to.

Take a few moments each morning, to simply breathe. Expand, explore, enjoy. There is a reason that the breath is described as inspiration.

• • •

Take a moment to write down your answers to these questions:

How can you incorporate a few moments of gently breathing stretches into your daily routine?

_____

_____

_____

How relaxed can you stay as you try these exercises?

_____

_____

_____

How do you feel after five minutes of gentle easy breathing?

_____

_____

_____

What personal strengths have you had to draw on to create this daily routine?

_____

_____

_____

15

Joe: Moving Forward

Even though some mornings were tough, Joe still went to pulmonary rehab; they were expecting him. And, they always seemed happy to see him. Funny, he always felt better after he went.

They had recently begun a 'walk for wellness' competition amongst the rehab classes. The destination was Washington DC, several hundred miles away. The staff had placed a large map of the US on the far wall with different sets of push pins for each team. Joe's team was red and they decided to name their team the 'Red Barons'. Joe thought it was a little silly at first, thinking how could they ever walk that far in just six weeks, but people were getting pretty excited, especially when the other team inched ahead of them on the map. Keeping track of his walking time was easy as Ell kept him diligent about his walking schedule each day at home. He was up to ten minutes twice a day so far, and compared to others, he felt pretty darn good about himself. Down the hallway, through the living-room, across the dining room to the kitchen, back down the hallway to the bedroom. He was getting to where he didn't have to stop and rest that often anymore.

Their team was ahead this week, but the Screaming Eagles were right behind them. "We have to get a jump on them for next week," someone commented, "if we want to win this thing." "I'm planning on doubling my time next week, that will help." "I slacked off this week, but next week, I'll get some walking in for sure." "We just need to keep up our steady progress" "We need to do maybe just a little more." The team was psyched up. It was infectious. Joe felt part of the team and it made him feel good. He noticed others being impressed with his steady numbers on the tally sheet. He also noticed how some others did so much more than him. But he was doing his part, getting his team closer to their goal. He had missed only one day in the past two weeks. That was the day that he had two appointments and he was too exhausted after that to do much of anything.

He knew he was starting to get better; he was hoping that he would continue to improve like this until he regained some real independence. His funk was slowly lifting, even at home. He had fixed the light in the hall and he had changed the broken lock. "Two of my goals," he remembered, with a proud nod. That took a lot out of him, though. The bending and reaching was a challenge and he found he wasn't as excited about it as he thought he would be. "It's a good start, though." He thought. Ellie had him dressing and shaving every day and folding laundry which, although he wasn't crazy about it, actually made him feel more of a team partner and less like a victim.

Joe had finally gotten a little more routine to his day though it still took him a long time to get up and ready in the morning. Someone had mentioned slip on shoes instead of sneakers and he found it had helped save him some energy. He would get so out of breath just bending over to tie his shoes. Joe had started leaving the wheelchair at home when he came to class. It was a hike for him and some days he wasn't sure if he had it in him. After parking, Ellie would take his oxygen and he would walk the couple hundred feet to the elevator, and then from the elevator it was another hundred and fifty feet to the class. He rested in the waiting room for five minutes before going in to the gym. Sandy noticed at the end of the class and had asked him about it. "I walked," Joe said. Sandy's eyes widened and her smile broadened. "I knew you could do it, Joe! I'm so proud of you! You are getting better and better!" Joe blushed, feeling like a schoolboy.

Joe kept his ears open when Sandy or Mary started the discussions during class. He was getting some good ideas on how to make his life a little more livable. The pursed lip breathing was helping and so were some of the tips he had learned in the class about using his energy wisely and staying healthy.

He was getting edgy now that he had a little more energy and motivation and he wasn't content to stay home all the time. Joe's appetite seemed to come back too, which Ellie was thrilled about; he had lost so much weight. Joe started venturing out of the house, a little, out to lunch with Ellie or out shopping to the supermarket where he could use the electric cart. It was different though, being out; he had to carry that concentrator still wherever he went and he had slowed down a lot. But he noticed things more, like how serene the back yard felt just to sit on the patio, and how colorful the sunset was in the evening. He noticed people too, how they reacted to him in his wheelchair with his oxygen. He simply smiled and said good morning or some such greeting. Some days he tried to go out without his wheelchair. His distances were getting longer and he felt more confident on his feet. On the days he tried to do too much, he found that the following day he paid for it, and he had to struggle to get moving. But slowly, it was all coming together. "It won't be long now before I start taking walks to the park across the street." He thought, "I can picture it."

Take a moment to consider your answers to these questions:

What actions have you taken so far to reach your goals?

_____

_____

_____

How does achieving your goals make you feel?

_____

_____

_____

What's been the hardest part of your work so far towards your goal?

_____

_____

_____

What personal strengths have you had to draw on to get this far?

_____

_____

_____

16

Medicines and O2

When I fell, you helped me back up.

Medication can be dangerous and should never be taken lightly. And yet, medicine can be vital to our health. Do you know that medication errors are the third most common cause of death in the US? Be aware of what you are taking, why you are taking it, and how your medicines are affecting you. Errors can occur by the person taking the medicine, the pharmacist who dispenses them, the nurse who administers them, and by the physician who prescribes them. So be aware. You are the one at risk.

Having good communication with your doctor is a priority. Your doctor suggests, advises, explains, and prescribes. But you are the one who actually self-administers the medication. So, understand what to expect and what to watch out for. If you don't feel any better after taking a medicine or if there seems to be no positive impact on your health and well-being, ask your doctor if it is important enough to continue and why.

The average person in this country takes seven drugs. Are they all necessary? Ask your doctor at least twice a year and maybe check with the pharmacist. Do you really need to keep taking each of those drugs? Although you don't necessarily notice a difference in the way you feel, it may be keeping your lab numbers in the normal range or possibly preventing complications.

But maybe... Maybe ten years ago the doctor prescribed something for your sore toe and you continue to take it when it really isn't necessary.

Connect with your pharmacist. The pharmacist will explain what to expect, and when to notify the doctor of an adverse reaction.

The insert included with each prescription will describe medication-related information in more detail. Do you want to read the entire insert? Some people tend to be highly suggestible. If you read all the possible side effects and complications, will you suddenly start feeling those same effects?

And what about those over the counter drugs, supplements, vitamins? They are important too. They can impact how those prescribed medicines will work. The pharmacist's job is to assess any possible interactions that might be harmful. Use your pharmacist. Take advantage of that knowledge. Ask questions. Be sure that the pharmacist is aware of all of the medicines that you take, including the ones without prescription. Supplements and vitamins are included and can impact the effect of your prescribed medication and impact your health.

Know how to self-administer your drugs. If you use an inhaler, it is vital that you use it effectively so that the medication gets absorbed. Some people just do not have the power to inhale strongly enough and the effect of a medication is lost. Many have difficulty coordinating the inhalation with the compression of the vial and they lose most of the drug, absorbing little. I've run across so many clients who would say "These inhalers just don't do anything for me." When I ask them to demonstrate how they take the inhaler, it is clear that they simply don't absorb any of the drug. The drug ends up in their mouth and not in their respiratory tract where it does the work. A spacer is the best way to ensure that you are absorbing the entire dose. It allows you to compress the drug into the chamber and then inhale at your pace. You get the best bang for your breath using the spacer.

After inserting your medication into the device, detach the cover from the mouthpiece. Sit straight up (slouching inhibits your ability to inhale), slightly tilt your head back and exhale all your air, put the mouthpiece in your mouth, press the inhaler once and inhale slowly and deeply. Then, hold your breath for as long as you comfortably can. If it is a two-puffer medicine (like Albuterol) repeat this process again. But wait a minute or two after your first puff. Your bronchial tree will have a chance to absorb the initial dose, and start opening up. This will allow your second puff to go down deeper into your airway and have more effect. When taking a nebulizer treatment, again, sit up straight, relax, and breathe easy, every minute taking a deeper breath to allow the medicine to delve deeper into your lungs. It usually takes about 10 minutes to absorb all the medicine in the nebulizer. Take your time, relax and breathe. This is your time to imagine the drug opening your lungs, healing them, and easing your work of breathing.

After using your nebulizer be sure to wash it out well and air dry it. You don't want to re infect yourself or create an environment for mold or bacteria to grow.

There are lots of options for inhalers and nebulizer medications which are effective in opening up those tight and inflamed bronchial tubes.

Some bronchodilators work quickly and some work over a longer period of time. Some reduce inflammation. Some relax the tightness. It's a standard recommendation to be on a short acting as well as one or two long acting bronchodilators, possibly to include a steroidal inhaler to keep you breathing easy. Some inhalers are combinations. If more than one inhaler is prescribed at the same time, take the short acting inhaler first so that your bronchial tree will be wide open for the next, long acting inhaler. Remember, you are in charge of your body. Be sure to do your research online and then discuss the value and drawbacks of prescribed medication with your doctor.

Don't forget to rinse out your mouth after taking your inhalers, especially after the steroid inhalers. Residue from the inhaler is not meant for your gums or your healthy white teeth. Residue can cause an uncomfortable fungal infection in your mouth which is hard to get rid of and requires antifungal rinses over an extended period of time. Better to simply rinse and spit after using any and all your inhalers so there is no residue from any inhaler in your mouth.

If you have problems with any of your drugs, let the doctor know right away. If one doesn't agree with your stomach or your throat, let your doctor know; there may be an alternative that might work a bit better for you. Everyone responds differently to a medication. Listen to your body. Talk to your doctor. Tell your physician at each visit exactly how well or not well you are breathing, and how often you are using your short acting or rescue inhaler.

There are loads of new and better medications coming on board. Which one is right for you? Be aware, though that some medications build up over a longer period of time, so even if you don't feel a difference after taking it, sometimes in a week, you find you are breathing a little easier.

Exacerbations, or sudden worsening of your breathing can often be related to GERD, gastro esophageal reflux disease. This is when you regurgitate, often unknowingly, while sleeping at night. Inhalation of some of the contents of your stomach into your lungs causes inflammation and sometimes pneumonia. People with GERD have more frequent episodes of exacerbation, lung inflammation which leads to worsening lung damage. Avoid lying down right after eating. Try eating smaller meals. Spicy meals, or carbonated or alcoholic beverages may be causing some episodes of GERD. Ask your doctor if you might be safer taking an inhibitor or blocker to prevent this from occurring.

Harry was from Connecticut. He was prone to exacerbations, an inflammation in the lungs which landed him in the hospital fairly frequently. Harry started pulmonary rehab reluctantly, conceding that maybe, not likely, but maybe, he would notice a difference, if it didn't make him worse. He really didn't think that things would change but he accessed that hero inside of him. Harry soon realized that he had been comfortably complacent with his melancholy lifestyle. Did he really want to change? Rehab would get him up and going again. Yes, okay, he was going to do it. He started working on the treadmill for one minute at a time. Each week he would increase by one minute. In several weeks, Harry was on the treadmill for 10 minutes and feeling good, He increased the speed a bit continuing to increase his minutes bit by bit. Harry felt great. It was inspiring to see him quietly stick with his plan. He was steadily improving, doing 15 minutes on the treadmill at 1.5 mph. His wife, Connie, was thrilled to see the change in this man who, a few months ago, had thought his life was over. Connie came and watched each time, encouraging him on. She had such faith in Harry.

Unexpectedly, Harry had another exacerbation which brought him back to zero. After two weeks in the hospital, Harry came home and it was another two weeks before he returned to rehab. Again, Harry started on the treadmill, this time at 30 seconds. He was exhausted. But he kept on, confident that he would improve. Harry built himself up once again, never uttering a depressing word, always upbeat. "It wasn't easy, especially in the beginning, but I knew that it was the only way to get stronger. I was going to do it or not get better; it was all up to me. I'm not going to allow myself to give up again." He had too much to do. He and Connie had planned a vacation with family and he was going. Adding a minute more each week, he rebuilt his muscles and regained his breathing until he was on the treadmill once again for 15 minutes.

Harry had had some problems with some of the new medicines that the doctor had prescribed. They just didn't seem to be doing much. Someone in the support group mentioned a medication that had been working well for them and Harry brought the suggestion to his doctor. Harry and Connie went on vacation visiting family for a while. When they returned from vacation, they both stopped in to say goodbye to everyone in rehab. They were heading back to their home in Michigan. The new medication was working and he was feeling better than ever! He had stayed healthy with no setbacks since getting this new medication. He promised to continue his exercises daily. With that new medicine on board, Harry was feeling better than he had for years.

If your medication doesn't seem to be helping much, keep looking, asking, exploring.

Sometimes, injured alveoli have difficulty absorbing inhaled oxygen into the bloodstream, especially when you are exerting yourself, and your body is demanding more oxygen than usual. By increasing the percentage of oxygen available to your alveoli, either through the use of compressed gas or a device called a concentrator, you have more being absorbed into your system.

There are a variety of different oxygen concentrators out there. A concentrator is simply a device that pulls the oxygen from the air increasing the percentage from 21% to as high as 86 to 94%. You probably have a larger concentrator to use while you are home. Just a few things to be aware of:

▸ Keep the humidifier of the concentrator filled with distilled water so that your mouth and sinuses don't dry out.

▸ Remember to change the filter every year and a half.

▸ Replace your canula once monthly and the tubing at least once yearly.

▸ Be sure not to have open flames near your concentrator, as oxygen is flammable.

▸ Notify your power company if you are using oxygen. If there is ever a power outage, your home will be flagged to resume power before any others. In our town, the power company provides monthly discounts on your bill if you provide documentation from your doctor.

For going out and traveling, you will need something more portable. Condensed gas cylinders work well for many who are on high continuous flow. They come in different sizes from three to 10 pounds.

There are a huge variety of portable concentrator devices out there ranging from small two to three lb. machines to nine lb. machines. Although they are often carried on the shoulders, many prefer rolling carts that are easy to move about without having to carry a backpack, burdening the shoulders. Which oxygen concentrator is right for you depends on a lot of different factors: how much oxygen you use, how often you use it, how much it weighs, how much it costs, how durable it is and how long it lasts on battery. Some are continuous and some are pulse. Some are approved for airline travel and some are not. Most can be plugged into the car's DC outlet or cigarette lighter so you are not using the unit's battery. Many times, clients arrive at pulmonary rehab with questions about the best oxygen concentrator to get. You are surrounded by experts who not only have done the research but actually have experienced how well they work.

Find an oxygen provider that is available to you when you need their help. Ask your support group who they might recommend.

Some doctors prescribe three different liter flows depending on your activity. When you are sleeping your breathing is shallow, so you may need more liters per minute. When you are active, up and about, you may need more as your body is using more oxygen. And finally, when you are relaxing, ask what liter flow you should maintain.

The oxymizer is a special canula that maximizes the oxygen availability. It's a bit more cumbersome but it decreases the liters of oxygen you need to use.

Craig was an artist whose art works were being sold regularly in high end shops and boutiques along the coast of California. He had been pretty depressed before starting pulmonary rehab. He was particularly frustrated at his decreasing endurance when creative inspiration urged him to work for hours on end. He just couldn't do it anymore. A few bad exacerbations further wounded his lungs. Because he would become breathless with any exertion, his treatment team increased his oxygen to the limit of six liters through his canula. It wasn't enough. So, he went to the mask. When exercising he used a mask and increased his oxygen to 10 liters per minute so that he would be able to keep his O2 levels above 88% while exercising. He worked hard on the nu-step and the ergometer and walked the track. He always showed up, rarely missing a class. As Craig began using the mask regularly, his energy seemed to improve along with his mood. He measured his progress not by comparing himself to the others in the gym, but by his own standards. Craig recognized that everyone is different and cannot be compared. In support group, one day, Craig, with his normally quiet, unpretentious air, shared his feelings. "I am deeply and truly grateful for this oxygen cylinder. This tank allows me to continue to create, to work, to live. Without this tank, I wouldn't be here at all. I wouldn't be alive."

His sincerity struck the participants and awakened a new perspective. Yes, this tank, this albatross, that burdens you down wherever you go and whatever you do is something to appreciate.

• • •

Take a moment to write down your answers to these questions:

How up to date is your medication list and how often do you review this list with each of your doctors?

_____

_____

_____

_____

How confident are you at raising questions and concerns with your doctor?

_____

_____

_____

_____

What actions can you take to be your own best advocate?

_____

_____

_____

_____

17

Stress Management

"What we think determines what happens to us, so if we want to change our lives, we need to stretch our minds." —Wayne Dyer

S tress is a normal natural aspect of life. Everyone has stress and everyone copes with it differently, some more effectively than others. Some people swallow their stress, until it starts ebbing out into hypertension, increased blood sugars, shortness of breath, headaches, insomnia, or depression. The long-term effects are vast and innumerable, affecting our physical well-being along with our mental and emotional health.

You will always have stress in your life. From the moment you wake and the alarm clock goes off, your stress levels are increasing. You feel the urgency of getting up and getting out to work or to your appointments. Maybe you turn on the morning news and hear about the recent gun violence, the political intrigue and the drop in the DOW and your stress levels once again increase. You down a couple of cups of coffee, speeding up your metabolism. Your mind starts rolling on the worries of the day. Then, you get into the car and roll into traffic. Cars are jamming and honking as you realize you will be late. Cortisol is pouring into your bloodstream increasing blood pressure, heart rate, tightening muscles and slowing your immune system. Blood sugar rises as sugar is released from your liver; with nowhere to go it sits there a while straining your insulin pump until finally it turns into abdominal fat. Life in America. Sound familiar? That's just the beginning of course.

The events, themselves do not create stress. Stress comes from how you perceive these events. In other words, it's all in your mind. Your mind is a powerful tool that can either help you or hurt you depending on how you decide to use it or control it.

Stress can be effective sometimes when it is short lived. If we are faced with a sudden challenge, like exercise or a test, acute stress strengthens our muscles, sharpens our senses, and heightens our focus.

Chronic stress comes from the worries, fears and anxieties that plague thoughts causing eventual breakdown and illness. Its estimated that 90% of illness and injuries are chronic stress related.

So how do you manage stress?
First, you need a strong defense.

Sleep: 7 to 8 hours a night gives your body the stamina it needs to get through the day.

Good food: Real food. Living on twinkies, doughnuts, and fries puts a strain on your energy and your stamina.

Exercise: The number one best stress reliever, depression reliever, invigorator and self-esteem enhancer. Taking a walk each day in nature calms down a scattered mind. If you feel unable to walk, put some music on and sway. Simply move.

Support and connection: The healthiest population tend to be those who have connections with others. Today's world is becoming increasingly isolated as we close down in front of computers and smart phones. Reconnect with friends and loved ones. Make the first move. Who would you call if you needed help? If you are not sure, this indicates that maybe you are not there for support. Go find someone to support. This does not require financial or physical effort. A simple phone call sends the message. A hug, a note of appreciation, or simply showing interest can send a powerful message.

What do you stress about? Are they things you have control over? Or not? Are you waiting for the cheese to re-appear? Move on. Be realistic. No one can usually accomplish the same things they could twenty years ago. So, what. You can do other things.

Most identify their biggest stressors as finances, relationships, illness, or injury. One of my clients actually became so agitated when he watched the news that he had a heart attack. Was it worth it? Did it change anything? Only himself and his heart.

Remember the 4 A's of stress management:

Avoid the stressor — Learn how to say no, avoid people who stress you out. Control your environment. Cut down your "to do" list to only "must do's" and stop watching the news. Watch a comedy instead. You know the saying: 'Laughter is the best medicine'. It's true. Research has shown it to be very effective in healing the body and the mind.

Alter the stressor — Express your feelings, be willing to compromise. Be more assertive, manage your time better. If you are worried about being late, prepare the night before and wake up fifteen minutes earlier.

Adapt to the stressor — Look at your problems in a different way. Focus on the positive. Is there something you might change in yourself that will make things go a little easier? Take a less congested though maybe a little longer route to your appointments and enjoy the ride.

Accept the stressor — Don't try to control the uncontrollable. Look for the upside, share your feelings. Learn to forgive. If you can't get your husband to do something you want, see the good things he does that you maybe hadn't noticed before. Appreciate that and tell him that you appreciate that. He may just turn around and be more likely to want to make you happy.

What is the impact of anxiety, tension and worry on breathing? HUGE! Anxiety starts in your mind. 'I can't make it....', 'I'm worried about....', or, 'what if......'. Thoughts grow like parasites in the back of your mind seeping into your chest muscles, and your respiratory muscles, your bronchial tree and your shoulders. Everything tightens until you feel like you are trying to breathe with a vice squeezing your chest. You feel you can't catch your breath. As you focus on the tightness, you become more tense, further tightening those breathing muscles. Anxiety increases as the tension and shortness of breath increases, and the cycle continues. This is called the dyspnea cycle. It is uncomfortable and frightening. How do you stop it? Pursed lip breathing. Stop, rest, focus on breathing slowly, easily and gently. Slow, easy breaths in, gentle long easy breaths out. Focusing on your breath has been a meditation method used for centuries by monks to quiet the mind which quiets the body.

Dr. Woods shares that sometimes he sees young, healthy people in his office complaining of shortness of breath and chest pain. "These kids have become so anxious; it takes their breath away. They truly can't breathe but it needs to be treated with stress management tools, not drugs." Anger, fear and worry cost you, no one else.

In yoga, breathing has been found to be a powerful anecdote for calming a busy, stressed out mind.

Guilt and shame are deadly toxins. Thinking that we're somehow bad, that we are responsible for our illness helps nothing, least of all our bodies and can further be interpreted by our bodies as a desire for the body not to work well, because you don't feel that you deserve to be well. If you are harboring grief for times lost, mistakes made, or difficulties encountered in the past, it is time to identify the guilt and let them go. Write them down and destroy them. Accept, allow, and release them.

There was an Indian woman who had lost her brother in a terrible accident a few years ago and since then, had developed an excruciating pain in her right shoulder that debilitated her to the point where she was unable to walk upright. Doctors were at a loss to help her; no pain reliever or surgery could reduce the pain. Finally, she asked the medicine man in her tribe for help. He looked at her with compassion and asked, "Why are you still carrying your brother on your shoulder. It is long past time to let him go." She suddenly recognized the painful burden of guilt she carried when her brother had died. He had been her little brother and she felt responsible for his death. She decided to release her guilt, let it go, and her pain was lifted.

Depression is the lack of all energy and emotion, the lack of interest in life. 'What's the point?' 'Why try?' Too tired, too much work, no energy, no interest, no motivation, no appetite. Depression can and does happen to everyone from time to time. But be aware. If it is not moving out after a couple of weeks, it's time to take action. If exercise, support group, and your pet dog can't pull you back into the spirit of living, consider asking your doctor if you might need an antidepressant for a while, to jump-start you back into life. This doesn't mean it's forever, but it can give you the boost to start moving again.

If you notice the tension building, especially in your chest, here are some ways to reduce the anxiety.

Guided Imagery is used to demonstrate the amazing power the mind has over the body. Sit quietly and imagine yourself sitting by a rippling blue stream under the maple trees. The sun feels warm on your face and the forest opens up on the other side to a field full of wildflowers. Listen to the stream, watch the flow of the water bouncing over rocks in its bed. Feel the brush of the wind in your hair, see the glow of the sun reflect off the leaves. Allow yourself to sit and enjoy this experience for five minutes. Guided imagery is based on the concept that your body and mind are connected. Using all of your senses, your body seems to respond as though what you are imagining is real. Your heartbeat slows, your muscles relax, your breathing eases. You feel content.

**Try this simple breathing technique next time
you are beginning to feel anxious:**

- Breathe in for the count of 5

- Hold this breath for the count of 5

- Slowly exhale for a count of 5

- Hold for the count of 5

- Repeat

Journaling: Express the worry, fears, regrets, guilt and let it go. Close the chapter and move on. Start writing the next chapter, however you would like it to be.

Walk: Exercise distracts the mind, expels the pent-up energy produced in the body and makes you feel better.

Get a pet or volunteer at a pet shelter. Find someone who needs support: Sometimes when we focus our attention on ourselves, we get more tense and more aware of every nook and cranny of pain. A pet grabs your attention and has needs only you can take care of.

Get engaged in something or with someone outside yourself.

Mindful meditation is a strategy that controls the mind by focusing on the moment, right now, the sights the sounds, the smells the feel. There is only this, the here and the now. Everything else is in our heads.

Still having a problem? Try reflexology, chiropractice, or acupuncture. Naturopathic remedies. A soothing herbal tea, easy music, coloring, or sculpting.

Several years ago, I went to see a fortune teller, as I was terribly worried and concerned about several issues occurring in my life. My son was dealing with serious health issues, my finances were in bad shape, and my relationship was deteriorating. "$20" she said. I scraped my bag for a twenty but came up short. "What can I get for a ten?" I asked. She sighed. "Okay. Sit down. Think of three things you are concerned about." I had no trouble with this task as these issues were taxing my mind constantly. She took my hand in hers, opened it and looked at it closely, examining the lines that crisscrossed my palm. She closed her eyes. After a few moments had passed, she looked up and gazed into my eyes. "Everything will be just fine."

I never worried about those issues again. I never had the need to see another fortune teller. And, yes, everything turned out fine. Find yourself that fortune teller and you will be all set. You'll be counting your blessings daily!

Jeff was a 40-year-old construction engineer who was confronted with severe lung problems several years ago. The reason, like so for many others, was unknown, a virus, maybe, or simply a genetic fluke. But life moved on and so did he. He had to stop working but he was determined he wouldn't stop living. "Some people with lung issues seem to be waiting for the other shoe to drop, the hiccup that causes life to fall apart. We all need to live it now. Since being diagnosed, my dream of skydiving was dashed. So, I changed direction and started planning other things that I had wanted to try. I've always loved music and took classes in sound engineering. I'm now doing sound for a rock band in town, they're a great bunch of guys; we have fun."

By releasing the worry, and redirecting your thoughts to see the blessings, you open your airways and breathe easier. The heart and lungs work better and the immune system functions much more efficiently so you can fend off infections. And the bonus is that you feel happy!

• • •

Take a moment to write down your answers to these questions:

What is the cause of your stress?

_____

_____

_____

Can you change the situation? How?

_____

_____

_____

Can you change yourself? How?

_____

_____

_____

What could help you to feel better?

_____

_____

_____

18

Joe and Ellie: Reconnecting

"The most important thing in life is to learn how to give out love, and to let it come in." —Morrie Schwartz, author of *Tuesdays with Morrie*

J oe stayed true to his promise and arrived at rehab each Tuesday and Thursday at 11. Ellie would sit in the waiting room with other husbands and wives. Ellie found it helpful to have the opportunity to learn how others were coping with this burden. No one found it easy. Some had it much harder than her. And it felt reassuring to know that she was not alone in her trials. She picked up some good tips on how to make life a little easier for them both at home. She realized how much she had needed support. Ellie had always been the quiet, steady, follow-things-through person for Joe. But she had grown tired and disconnected lately. Ellie felt unappreciated and it seemed that the more she tried to help and support, the more he seemed to resent her. These husbands, wives, siblings, and children surely must have feelings like that sometimes, she thought.

Once a month, Joe and Ellie stayed for the support group where the agenda might include discussions with a pulmonologist, a pharmacist, a dietician, or a representative from an oxygen provider. Sometimes they learned about mindfulness meditation or reiki. Mostly, the agenda centered on what medicines worked best, or what lozenges to take to keep your mouth from drying. They learned about the latest new gadgets. Once in a while, they just talked. They talked about feelings but Ellie never brought up how she felt about their life at home. She wondered how many of the family members there had feelings similar to her own. Unappreciated, taken for granted.... "But that is just selfish of me to even think about it," she thought. "It's so hard for him and all I can do is feel bad for myself." She admonished herself for her self-pity and she tried to brush it off. At one particular meeting, though, they had a counselor speaking. The counselor talked a little about relationships and coping and then he asked the group to share. Ellie tried to think of some way she could broach the subject when Cindy, one of the other wives, mentioned some of her frustrations at home. She said that sometimes Alan didn't seem to respect her anymore. Cindy looked at Alan with a smile and grabbed his hand. "I love him and want the best for him, but I feel sometimes that I am losing myself completely. We just don't seem to connect anymore." The therapist nodded. People started talking more about what matters in a relationship and how sometimes people get so lost in their own world, it's easy to forget what really matters.

Joe and Ellie always walked away from these meetings feeling hopeful. They had both learned so much and felt a bond with the other couples in the group. Joe was improving, getting stronger, feeling more engaged in life. This meeting had given Ellie the courage. She knew it was time to talk to Joe about her feelings.

When they went home that night, they sat down at the kitchen table with their tea and they talked. Ellie, first, shared how much she loved Joe and how desperately she wanted to maintain that close bond that they had in the past. She opened up about her frustrations, and how she just didn't know how to get the old Joe back, the Joe she had married. Joe listened quietly, nodding his head and looking at her with tenderness and understanding. "I know, it's been hell for you, Joe, and maybe I'm being selfish even to bring this up." Joe smiled, kissed her. He admitted that he had been pretty stuck in his own anger since this situation happened. "I didn't even realize how selfish I'd been, Ell, just trying to get through each day. I think I got lost in my own head and wasn't thinking about how tough it might be for you. I love you and I appreciate what you do for me. Let's talk about how we can make things work a little better."

They realized that they had a lot to be grateful about. Overall, life was getting better. Both looked at each other with compassion and love. They came up with some changes in their day that would help out the other, like starting with a morning hug and helping out with some chores. Joe recognized that he didn't need Ell to get his medicines ready, he could do it himself, now. Joe decided secretly that he would get her coffee ready in the morning; he knew that would make her feel appreciated. It's a start. When they finished their tea, Ellie and Joe headed for the bedroom. "Let's try, I know it's been so long. I'll take my inhaler, boost up my oxygen a bit and we'll take it slow. I love you so much, Ellie. I want to feel close to you again. I've missed you." Ellie smiled and kissed Joe softly, holding him close. "We can take it slow and easy. Just promise to talk to me. Let me know how you are doing, how we can make this work."

Relationships are never easy. There is an ebb and flow to the day to day interactions between couples. Without noticing, unsaid feelings can grow and fester inside, stretching that once perfect bond. How do you stay close when crisis becomes chronic? Many people become so wrapped up in their own problems and activities that they forget the relationship; they forget that maybe what they said or did has been misinterpreted or misunderstood.

We all need to feel loved and capable. When these vital aspects of our identity become threatened, either at home or at work, we may, without even realizing it, express our pain by hurting the ones we love. We didn't mean to hurt them but we lash out at those we know will take it and probably not stop loving us.

Sometimes relationships die of boredom. We get hardened from the lack of response to our attempts to create closeness. We stop communicating. Feelings of frustration, anger, resentment build. We forget how to connect and we blame the other, sometimes without the other even realizing it.

Communication is vital to any relationship. But how do you open the doors to feelings without alienating each other in the process? You each want to be understood. You each want to understand. You recognize that there is no winner in your arguments, only losers. Maybe we simply forget that our first priority is understanding, appreciating and accepting the other's feelings. You want to make it work- because you love each other. That is the first priority.

Sometimes creating the time and place where you each feel safe is a start, having a time out when you don't feel safe, and by truly listening with the heart when honest feelings are shared. No one chooses to have feelings; they are simply there. Feelings are neither bad nor good. But once you are aware of how the other feels, perhaps together you can make simple changes towards more loving behaviors.

· · ·

Take a moment to write down your answers to these questions:

How do you show you care?

_____

_____

_____

How does your loved one share their feelings with you when they have a problem?

_____

_____

_____

How do you share your feelings with your loved one when you have a problem?

_____

_____

_____

How do you feel after your discussion?

_____

_____

_____

19

Seriously: Stop Smoking

You have faith in my ability to move forward.

If **you are smoking still, it is time to breathe and stop smoking.** There are lots of ways to do this. Ask your doctor and your team for help and suggestions. Get in touch with the American Lung Association in your region and ask them about classes. Find a support group or support person who will be there for you and talk you out of temptation. Having the support of a wife or husband, or even better, quitting together improves the health of you both. Make it a competition.

Get rid of ashtrays, lighters, and random cigarette packages. Make the decision and go cold turkey.

Change your routines which trigger you to smoke. Do you have one with your morning coffee? Do morning stretches first, eat breakfast then start another activity without stopping to light up. Try tea or a different drink, or try having your coffee in a different place.

Ashline is a volunteer group that supports your efforts to quit smoking by checking in with you once or twice a day to see how you're doing. They give you support and ideas, and keep you motivated.

Change habits; refocus your attention on something else. Change your eating patterns. Take up a hobby that engages your hands, knitting, crocheting, writing, playing guitar. Try singing, macramé, woodcraft, yoga, pet sitting, journaling. When you are using your hands, you are keeping your mind focused on something new and positive. Start walking immediately after breakfast. Get in shape and rediscover the person you can become. One friend and patient crotchets plastic bags, turning them into shopping bags for the homeless while she is sitting watching TV in the evening. Taking up a new hobby to replace the smoking habit refocuses your attention and moves your attention towards your new activity.

Recognize your weak moments and have a plan ready. Sometimes, people will have rubber bands wrapped on their wrist and when the urge strikes, they snap the rubber band which focuses their mind on the sting and reboots their thinking away from the urge. Snaps are counted up at the end of the day. You can gauge your progress from the decrease in your daily snaps.

Brush and whiten your teeth, and use mouthwash more often. Be sure to wash your clothes that smell like tobacco. Air out the house so that there's no evidence of tobacco odors.

Supplement your changes in activity with medication. This will double your stamina. Chantix has proven to be an effective tool in the quitting process, removing the physical craving. Others have found Wellbutrin to be helpful. Nicotine patches might be beneficial. Ask your team about these and other options.

There are those who were smoking two packs a day that were hypnotized and felt no need to smoke at all afterwards, experiencing no withdrawal difficulties at all.

Have carrot sticks, celery sticks, and maybe coffee stirrers available to satisfy the oral craving. Sugarless gum or hard candy will keep your mouth active.

Remind yourself continuously of how you are helping your lungs improve, how much better and lighter you feel, and how your family is staying healthier.

I was a smoker, and found myself sneaking cigarette breaks in the bathroom when the children were sleeping. When they discovered the packages of cigarettes, they would crush them and admonish me. I was embarrassed. I was the parent, but they knew better, and I recognized that. By the time they were six and four years old, I had stopped smoking. I knew that I was a role model for my children, I didn't ever want them to smoke cigarettes. But the effort was a slow, cigarette by cigarette process. Little by little I gradually erased the activity from my routines.

Find the method that works for you and do it. Forgive yourself; it is an integral part of getting better. Reacquaint yourself with your own potential and your gifts. Create a list of your strengths and focus on them daily. Write out your affirmation, "I am proud to be a nonsmoker!" and place it on your bathroom mirror where you see it several times a day.

Get up and get out. Get out of the chair frequently and connect with family friends and community. Do your share whatever that might be. Drying dishes, Folding clothes, dusting, fixing the clock, maintaining financial accounts. You are on the team that maintains the home.

Maybe it's one less cigarette a day until you stop or maybe it's cold turkey. Eventually you will succeed. If you fail at first, move forward and start again. Let go of the guilt and see yourself as a winner, a non-smoker. Energy will increase, breathing will be easier, coughing will be less, food will taste better, and you will look better.

• • •

Take a moment to write down your answers to these questions:

What are some ways you might consider trying to cut down on your smoking?

_____

_____

_____

_____

What resources can you call on to help you achieve your non-smoking goal?

_____

_____

_____

_____

What would be the benefits to you and to your family when you become a non-smoker?

_____

_____

_____

_____

20

The Elixir of Energy

"You may be going slow right now but you are still faster than everyone on the couch." —S. Lear

Delores came to pulmonary rehab because her doctor urged her to try it. She had been using a walker to get about, but lately she found that she just didn't have the energy for even that, so she started using the wheelchair more and more. "What do you do at home for activity, Delores, I asked? "Well, I knit, and I love to read, mmmm…and I watch TV. I have a lovely lazy boy lounge chair with my drinks and my medicines right next to me. I don't really get out much anymore, it's just too much work and I am so tired. My COPD is just getting worse."

"It's not necessarily your COPD that is the cause of your tiredness, but the lack of activity. You see, the less you move, the less you want to move. It becomes harder and harder until finally it's easier to use a wheelchair. Where do you go from there?"

"Last week," she said, "I was so embarrassed. I had stopped to use the toilet while I was shopping at the supermarket. I got out of the electric cart and got myself into the toilet okay. When I was finished, I couldn't get myself up off the toilet. I had to call out from the ladies' room for someone to come and help me. It was just so embarrassing." Delores's face turned red just remembering that day. That was the motivation Delores needed to get up and get moving. And she did. After working on some sit stand exercises using a pillow and initially two hands, she was able to use only one hand and finally she strengthened her legs enough to stand without using her hands at all. She was delighted. An interesting thing is that she tended to get out more, to the mall and to restaurants with friends. She was walking more, storing her wheelchair in the garage for use on longer outings only. Her confidence as well as her stamina had improved immensely.

Remember, you have over 600 muscles in your body and if you don't use them, you lose them. They shrink and shrink until you can't stretch them out. Have you ever noticed how you get up out of your chair these days? Do you jump up on your feet without thinking, like you did when you were a child or do you brace your hands on the armrest and push yourself up? It's a good idea to work on standing up and sitting down without using your hands. This might be a gradual process, starting with both hands then eventually, one hand, until you are using only your legs. Be sure you are leaning forward with your butt on the front half of the chair, and the back of your legs touching the edge of the chair. Lean forward and as you exhale, push up. This strengthens your leg muscles, improves your balance and keeps you strong and independent.

Exercise doesn't have to be difficult or time consuming. Walking and stretching simply keeps you flexible, able to get up out of bed easier. It strengthens your muscles and bones so you can pick up some groceries and move them. It gives you the endurance to walk from your car into the movie theatre or concert seats. Sure, COPD tends to slow down your pace a bit, but with exercise, pausing, pursed lip breathing, and pacing, you can do it.

Thirty minutes of moving each day, as study after study found, will improve your heart and lungs, your blood pressure, your blood sugar, your outlook, your muscles and joints; it will improve your ability to move, lift, and stretch. You will be happier, have more energy and think more clearly. You will sleep better, be more regular, and connect with others more. The list continues. If doctors could give you a pill that could provide all that, how much would you pay? And yet, it can be yours with a half hour each day. People have been able to stop taking their pills for their diabetes and their high blood pressure medications completely after a few improvements with diet and exercise. The key is getting motivated enough to actually do it.

Break it up during your day, five minutes, six times a day, or ten minutes after every meal. Turn the music on and dance while you are house cleaning. That counts! Invest in a portable peddler and pedal while watching TV. There are lots of ways to get 30 minutes of movement that can be fun and rewarding. Plan a short walk with a friend, first thing in the morning. Knowing that someone is waiting for you is a sure motivator to get you up and moving.

Exercise includes keeping your joints loose and easy. A few minutes of stretching can allow you to get in and out of your car with ease, bend over to grab your shoes, twist to see who is behind you while driving and stay balanced when you lift your foot, reach over or up into the cabinet.

Before getting out of bed, in the morning stretch your arms and legs out as much as you can, then squeeze together, roll your head from side to side. Stretch your toes forward, then all the way back. Pull your arm across your body, one arm at a time. Clench, then stretch out your fingers. Swing your arms up and around in a circle. When you are up, swing your arms from side to side, bend sideways, as you are standing, from side to side. Lower your head to one side then the other.

Strength gives you the power to lift, to stand up, to push and pull. All those little things you take for granted when you are younger. Grab two cans of soup from your cupboard. Lift the cans from your shoulder level in front of you up then down back to shoulder level, lift them forward in front of you, then lower them. Lift them out to the side then down. Bend your elbows up, bringing the cans up to the level of your shoulders, then down. Start slow, maybe three or four times, and increase the number of times that you do each of these exercises until you reach fifteen. Then find bigger cans.

Endurance lets you go further and longer with ease. That's where a walking program works great. Start small and increase in increments that keep you slightly challenged but still feeling good about it. By gradually increasing the amount of time, the frequency, the intensity of your work out you will feel lighter, brighter and more confident.

Pamela could walk only fifty steps when we started our Walking for Wellness competition. By the end of the competition, six weeks later she had improved her walking to twenty minutes a day. She was elated. "My breathing is so much better and my phlegm seems to clear out more easily. My husband takes my oxygen and we walk to the end of the street and back. We take our time and I stop if I need to. He told me I had so much more color in my cheeks and that I look even more beautiful! He is proud of me I know." Pamela was glowing.

Sure, you were able to do all those things a few years ago without exercising at all. As you get older, muscle mass shrinks much more quickly. Just a few days in bed without moving and your muscles are stiff, weak and tired. Luckily, if you have been an exerciser, your muscles remember quickly and seem to recover more quickly.

Pulmonary rehab staff can help you set up a safe individualized program that will meet your own personal goals. If there is no pulmonary rehab near you, start slowly, maybe walking a minute or two minutes. If you become out of breath or fatigued, or if your oxygen levels drop, stop, rest, breathe, then continue. This is not a race. If your oxygen level continues to drop below 88%, your doctor will probably suggest that you bump up your oxygen a liter higher than normal. Just turn it down when you have completed your exercise. After completing your one minute, or your three minutes, give yourself a pat on the back! Good job! Gradually increase your time walking little by little, minute by minute until you are walking for 30 minutes a day.

Remember, listen to your body. Every day may be different. If it is easy, and your numbers are fine, ramp up, do more, either by increasing the time, the frequency, or the intensity of what you are doing. If it is exhausting or if it feels really hard, turn it down. Your goal is to exercise at a place where you feel you are working but not to the point of exhaustion or pain. Be smart. Watch your oxygen. If you are smiling at the end, good.

Tune in to your breathing and exertion. Don't tax yourself out for the rest of the day. If you do that, it's too much. You should feel good with what you accomplish. This is not a fight to the finish. Slow and easy. Remember the tortoise! Pursed lip breathing with your exercise improves performance and increases oxygen levels. Rome wasn't built in a day but step by step, you can get closer to your goal. Be patient with yourself.

George had been diagnosed with pulmonary fibrosis. He felt like there was really no point in attending the rehab program, but he promised his doctor that he would give it a try. His symptoms had been gradually increasing over the past few years and he was doing very little at home; computer games mostly, or TV. Just a couple of years previous, he had been arranging million-dollar sales with large corporations. George used to be gregarious and social but he changed. He rarely left home and when he did, he used the wheelchair when he had doctor's appointments and such. His wife, Jackie, was ever vigilant, working 24-7 to meet his every need. "You are a team," I asserted; "it's not fair, Jackie, that you do everything for him. George is capable of carrying out chores at home and if you don't allow him that responsibility he feels like an invalid." George's smile was flat. He confessed to feeling little joy in his life.

I asked him if he could be consistent with rehab for the first three weeks and if he found no relief from his symptoms, I wouldn't press him further. George had been an avid road biker. Since retiring two years ago, he had given up on any activities. But George, true to his word, put in the effort, and within a few weeks, found himself looking forward to seeing his new friends in rehab. Within a couple of months, he was riding the stationary bike at speeds faster than the others and his treadmill was on an incline. At home, he was tasked with the laundry, drying dishes, and some meal preps. He and his wife were going out more to visit friends and family and he started to go shopping with his wife without using the electric cart. "I just take my time, and hang on to the cart while I walk. That pursed lip breathing seems to help a lot." George wasn't keen on using the wheelchair as much anymore "When will you take your bike for a ride?" I asked. "Already have," he said. "I rode around the block with my oxygen in the basket. Not easy, but I felt great; my goal is to ride a mile." A smile erupted on his face, an authentic smile, and I could feel his sense of confidence and joy in life returning.

Base your exercise program on how you are feeling. This can change each day. On a day when you are having increased problems breathing or increased fatigue, it may be wise to decrease your exercise. Remember these tips:

► Do not exercise when you are ill.

► Drink water.

► If you feel chest pain, severe shortness of breath, sudden left arm, shoulder, jaw neck or back pain, dizziness, nausea, profuse sweating, or weakness, just stop and rest. If it does not improve after resting for two minutes, or it gets worse call 911.

Find the time of day that's right for you and stick by it. Get a routine. For me, first thing in the morning I stretch and lift. Later in the day, I walk or bike.

Exercise helps to take away those aches and pains and gives you vitality. And best of all. Its free, you can do it anywhere, and when done wisely, not overdoing, there are very few side effects and no complications! That's even better than medicine!

• • •

Take a moment to write down your answers to these questions:

What exercise program can you plan into your day?

_____

_____

_____

What times of day can you exercise?

_____

_____

_____

When can you start this program?

_____

_____

_____

How can you stay accountable to this plan?

_____

_____

_____

21

What are you Eating?

"If you keep good food in your fridge, you will
eat good food." —E. McAdams

Asian Ayurveda is an ancient healing practice that promotes balance of healing energies in the body. According to Ayurveda, there are three natural body types. Vatta people are thin, and are often higher strung, Pitta are usually more average size, more balanced. Kapha are broad boned, slower, gentler. Whichever you happen to be, accept it. Appreciate who you are. By eating the appropriate foods, you can keep your body in balance.

The food you eat may actually be one of the reasons you don't feel well. Indian medicine women treated illness and injury with herbs from the earth. Can food be considered medicine? That processed food, even though you may have been under the impression that it was healthy, may be causing you to have high blood pressure, diabetes, fatigue, headaches, bowel problems, and more. What you eat can either kill you or cure you.

A woman with terminal cancer decided to forgo the chemotherapy and try a nutritional treatment. She was advised to eat a large daily ration of beets. At her follow up visit, the doctor announced to her that the cancer was gone. Another friend was told that she needed a colectomy for her digestive issues. She decided to try eliminating gluten from her diet. Her digestive problems were gone.

We know the right food choices can improve diabetes, heart disease, and digestive disease. Maybe there are other effective nutritional treatments.

Some doctors at Kaiser Medical in California hand out recipes instead of prescriptions. Can food be helpful with your breathing? A study in Japan showed that kiwi fruit decreased the frequency of asthma attacks. Spicy food, such as foods with cayenne pepper, can open up your sinuses and respiratory tract.

Can food be a better cure than drugs?

Dr. Hyman at the Cleveland Clinic sees food as natural medicine. He says, "About 70 to 80% of your diet should be plant foods, like vegetables, whole grains, beans, and fruits." Remember the five a day rule? That's at least three servings of vegetables each day and two fruits. There is a reason that your grandmother advises, 'An apple a day keeps the doctor away.' Processed foods, anything that doesn't look like it came from the earth may not be your friend. If you can't understand the list of ingredients on the outside, it may not be real food. When grocery shopping, the more you can shop on the perimeter of the store, the less processed foods will make it into your cart. The key is to go simple and eat in moderation.

Be wary of the nitrates found in processed meats, hot dogs, bacon, and deli meats. They are known for exacerbating your COPD, progressing the disease process, and increasing your risk of lung cancer. Non nitrate meats are available in your supermarket. You just want to check the label.

High fructose corn syrup is a processed food. This ingredient is related to obesity, diabetes, and high blood pressure. Beware of its sneaky addition to the most unsuspecting foods: crackers, breads, yoghurts. It is empty sugar calories that can easily turn into fat around your middle.

Regular sugar is an oxidizer that creates inflammation. The inflammatory response produces swelling and increases phlegm in your airways. Anti-inflammatory foods, like salmon, tuna, broccoli, cauliflower, nuts, olive oil, strawberries, apples, blueberries, kiwi, and avocado are wonderful options. These can help keep your lungs and bronchial tree open and clear.

Are you underweight? You may be burning more calories just from the work of breathing than the number of calories you are taking in. Remember; calories in versus calories out. If you are too thin and need to gain weight try eating small amounts of high calorie foods six to eight times a day. Cashews, avocado, coconut, yams, yogurt, peanut butter, and oatmeal might be good options. Consider eating every two to three hours.

If you are overweight, there might be extra pressure on your lungs causing more difficulty breathing and more fatigue. Moving can be exhausting. It's tough to carry twenty-pound weights across a room. If you are carrying an extra forty to fifty pounds in body weight, try turning it into muscle, exercising more frequently, so it strengthens you. Add more lentils, beans, and vegetables to your diet.

Use a small plate, and make enough food to have leftovers. I enjoy making a big soup with lots of vegetables, beans, and lentils, and maybe some lean meat at the beginning of the week. Soup is a quick, easy, low calorie option and gives me delicious lunches for the entire week.

Donna was frustrated as she was working so hard to lose weight but couldn't seem to lose a pound. "I'm eating all the right foods, fruits, vegetables, and no fat, and very little bread or pasta, my favorite. When I get hungry, I'll eat an apple or two. Why aren't I losing weight?" But, unfortunately, Donna was eating about 10 to 12 apples a day. "Apples are a good food, but they have a lot of sugar in them. So, all that extra sugar turns into fat." Mary, the nurse replied. "It might work better to snack on other kinds of low sugar alternatives, like celery and hummus, or bell peppers and yoghurt with ranch seasoning. One apple a day is fine. Twelve is too many. Too many of one food is never the right choice. Balance and moderation are key." Donna's eyes lit up. "Oh dear, I thought I was being so smart!"

Do you sometimes feel bloated after eating a large meal or after eating gassy foods? Do you notice that you get more tired and maybe have some tougher breathing? Try cutting down on the foods that cause you gas and eat smaller meals. Smaller meals will put less pressure on your breathing muscles. Chew slowly and consciously and wear your oxygen.

You might ask your doctor to check your vitamin levels and your thyroid hormones to ensure that you are not deficient. A deficiency might be causing some of your fatigue.

Tune in to your body. Habits, especially bad habits are so easy to develop. I tend to not over analyze what I eat but work to be smart, avoiding fried, processed, starchy, and sugary foods.

When I asked Linda what her goals were when she started at pulmonary rehab she said, "I want to lose a hundred pounds."

I responded realistically. "That's a very big goal. Can we make it twenty pounds maybe?" She said, "Oh no, I can do it. I've done it before, and I know I can do it again." Linda was obese, weighing 340 pounds.

After only six weeks, she had lost 35 pounds. "How did you lose 35 pounds so quickly and smoothly?" I asked? "I ate small meals, three times a day, with lots of vegetables, lean meat and fish, no starchy foods, sugar, high fat, or fried foods. It can be done."

The food you eat can help to cure you or can make you worse. This is your opportunity to make a direct impact on your own health. Choose balance and enjoy your meals.

• • •

Take a moment to write down your answers to these questions:

What are your eating patterns?

_____

_____

_____

_____

Do your eating habits help you feel better or drain your energy?

_____

_____

_____

_____

What improvement could you make in what you buy and eat that would

help you towards becoming the person you envision?

_____

_____

_____

_____

22

Joe: Redesigning His World

"You are never too old to set another goal or to dream a new dream." —C.S. Lewis

Joe found himself looking forward to the twice weekly sessions in rehab. He always felt so much better after he went, even though sometimes it was tough, having to get up and out by 10:30 so he would be on time. Joe had his alarm set for eight so he wouldn't have to rush.

He learned to prepare everything the evening before, his clothes, his meds, his oxygen and his keys. He even prepared the coffee the night before so it would be ready for Ell. He wasn't a big coffee person, himself but he liked doing those little things for her; he knew it made her happy. He never had thought of doing those little things before; the little things that let her know he was thinking of her. He had been so wrapped up in his own morose world. Now, he liked to think of new ways to make her smile. He found his sense of humor coming back and he would toss out silly jokes to make her laugh. He loved seeing her face light up when she laughed.

In rehab, he had his routine down. He was up to 15 minutes on the treadmill, 12 minutes on the bike and 20 minutes on the NuStep at level 7, a pretty good pace, and he was proud of himself. He had to push himself on the machines, but he knew his limits. And every time was a little different; some days were harder than others. Some days, he could do more. He wanted to try the elliptical soon. "That would be his next goal," he thought. Joe felt good, better than good.

A few weeks ago, when Joe and Ell had their weekly 'share how you're feeling now' session, he had told her that he was ready to be a little more independent. "I'll do just fine, Ell. You don't have to coddle me anymore. It's so much easier to get around now with this new portable oxygen tank."

So, starting two weeks ago he started going to rehab without Ellie. He had met another one of his goals! Joe felt like he was finally putting his life back together. It felt great to be back behind the wheel after six months, feeling in control. "I didn't realize how much I missed driving, how much I missed just having control." The wheelchair was gathering dust in the garage these days. He'd notice it when he got into the car each morning. Today he paused, remembering those days. "Don't need you much anymore, old fella', just for the ball games. It's a long way to get from the parking lot to those bleachers. Eventually, maybe, I'll get there on my own." He nodded. "Way to go, Joe," he thought with a smile.

Joe felt at home when he walked into the gym and everyone looked up and said hello. The guys would have jokes and stories ready to share. Sandy always asked how Ellie was doing. "She's off to her yoga class this morning with her friends. I don't get why she would want to twist into a pretzel twice a week, but she loves it."

Mary, the nurse in Rehab mentioned that they were thinking of trying out a new Tai Chi program. "Research has proven it to be effective for people with lung problems and we have an instructor willing to come in and share some of the exercises once a week. Maybe we could do Tai Chi instead of our stretches one morning a week for 10 minutes so that everyone who wanted could try it." "Hey, that sounds interesting. I've heard about Tai Chi but not sure what it's about." "Me too, I'd like to try it." "I'm game. I'm not ready to twist into a pretzel like Ellie, though." One of the others laughed. "OK, then, let's try it out next week and see how it goes;" Mary suggested, "and don't worry. You won't have to do any pretzel moves. Actually, I've done Tai Chi and its very relaxing. I think you will like it."

Take a moment to write down your answers to these questions:

Have you noticed any positive changes in your life?

_____

_____

_____

How confident are you feeling about making changes and moving forward?

_____

_____

_____

What did it take to get you to make the first move?

_____

_____

_____

When and how do you choose what to do next?

_____

_____

_____

23

Simple Fixes for a Good Night's Sleep

"Don't expect to see a change if you don't make one." —K. Saunders

Every living being sleeps, flowers close their petals, ants stop working, birds perch on their respective limbs, even fish snuggle under their seaweed beds and close their eyes.

Sleep is vital to your well-being, Sleep affects your ability to think; it affects your digestion, your heart, and your ability to fight off infections; it affects your outlook and your memory. Studies show that obesity, diabetes, and high cholesterol are more prevalent among irregular sleepers. Lack of sleep results in injuries, car accidents, and falls because you are just not alert enough to notice the curb or the stop sign. If you are trying to lose weight, how frustrating when you do everything right, cut down on the sugar, exercise and follow the prescribed meal plan and you still can't lose. Maybe you are not sleeping. Feeling depressed and lethargic? Maybe you are not getting the required seven to eight hours a night. Do you tend to fall asleep while watching TV or after eating, while riding in the car or sitting in traffic? You need to investigate! This is vital to your quest for better health, better stamina, stronger lungs! You may need a sleep study to determine the cause.

How to Sleep....

Set a schedule. Go to bed and get out of bed on the same schedule every day. Go to bed at 11:00 and get up at 7:am Even if you are not tired at the scheduled time, go to bed! If you wake up early, stay in bed until the scheduled time. You are training your body and brain.

Buy fresh pillows and replace your worn-out mattress. It doesn't cost a lot for a new mattress. Amazon has great mattresses for a few hundred dollars.

Leave the TV and other electrical gadgets outside the bedroom. They tend to stimulate your brain. The electromagnetic waves excite the neurons preventing relaxation. Avoid Alcohol before sleeping.

Stay cool in a dark room. Having light blocking or black out shades will keep out the early morning sunshine and will keep you sleeping longer. Your body temperature naturally cools as your body prepares for sleeping. You reinforce your body's tendency to drift off by keeping the room cooler. The coolness also stimulates melatonin, the hormone that regulates our biological clock. Lower the thermostat for the night time. Still having difficulty? Raising your head up with a few pillows will help ease the work of breathing.

Agitated? Is your mind filled with thoughts, worries, agendas, regrets? Try the tighten and release strategy from your toes to your scalp. With each part of your body, starting with your toes, then your feet, your lower legs, your thighs, your back, your belly, your shoulders, hands, arms, neck, face, scalp, tighten for a count of ten and release, letting those muscles relax. Finally, tighten your whole body, then relax. This can release that tension that you have been holding in all day.

Still having trouble? Try the 5-5-5-5 box breath technique. Breathe in for the count of five, hold for the count of five, breathe out for the count of five, hold for a count of five. The focus on your breath distracts your brain.

There are some music tracks of ambient natural sounds that can lull people to sleep; sounds of the ocean surf, soft rain falling, or maybe a rippling brook with birdsong in the background. One troubled soul finally discovered a series of breathing sounds to follow that allowed him to drift off contentedly.

Get exercise during the day but not just before going to sleep.

Have a pre bedtime routine, a warm shower, cup of chamomile tea, warm milk and crackers, or read a book, preferably a boring book. Write down your thoughts and feelings in your journal. Tart cherry juice contains some natural melatonin and can help you have a more restful sleep.

And before slumbering down, remember the three best happenings of the day and feel gratitude.

Stan was a CEO at a large corporation in the city. I asked him, "How do you manage to sleep with all that pressure on your shoulders?" He shared with me that he used to have terrible insomnia. "I discovered a technique to allow me to leave it all at the office. When I'm ready to sleep I imagine myself walking down a long hallway with open doors along each side, each door representing each upcoming task and decision. As I walk down the hallway, I close each door along the way until I come to the end. My mind accepts this as a way to close my thoughts about work. My mind becomes quiet and I sleep."

• • •

Take a moment to write down your answers to these questions:

What is keeping you awake at night?

_____

_____

_____

What has your doctor recommended to improve your sleep?

_____

_____

_____

How can you change your habits to improve your sleep?

_____

_____

_____

How do you feel after a good night's sleep?

_____

_____

_____

24

Doctoring Yourself

"The secret of your future is hidden in your daily routine." —M. Murdoch

Doctors love information. And they are always very impressed, listening a little closer, when their patients rattle off specifics. Your doctor maybe sees you once monthly, if that. He will take your blood pressure, take your weight, assess your color and your breathing, and check your oximetry. In order to be your own physician, these things and more are some of the things you can monitor on your own. When you wake up in the morning, that's when you want to do your own personal check up. What will you check?

You get up, go to your bathroom, empty your bladder. Is your urine light or dark, cloudy or clear? Dark urine indicates that you may not be taking in enough fluids. Cloudy urine or pink urine indicates a possible infection. Any pain or sense of urgency? Are you urinating large amounts or small amounts?

Next, look at yourself in the mirror, how do you look? How's your color? Are you pale, dusky or pink? Are your eyes clear? Are your fingers pink? Squeeze your fingernail. Does it blanche and then turn pink in less than 3 seconds? Good. That indicates that you are getting enough oxygen. Just to be sure, check your oxygen saturation. If it's 89% or better, good. If its 100% you might want to turn down your oxygen. If its lower than normal, why? Make a note.

Take a breath. How's the breathing today? Same as usual, or are you a little short? Assess your energy level, same as yesterday or are you more fatigued? Any new pain anywhere? Sore throat? Chest tightness? Any cough? Is your phlegm clear or light gray as usual or is it green or yellow? Is it a different color than usual? Is it thicker or thinner? Is there more or less? Any pain? Where? Any chest pains? Does it get worse or the same while breathing in? Is that new? It might indicate a pocket of pneumonia or pleurisy, or costochondritis or maybe you have been exercising too hard. Contact the doctor today. Caution. Any deviation from normal is something to identify and note down. Got your notebook right there? Good.

Is your bowel activity normal for you? Constipation can lead to problems. Keep track of it. If you get constipated, try drinking more prune juice and other fluids and be sure to have an exercise program. If constipation is a regular problem, talk to your primary care doctor. Do you have diarrhea? Be sure to replace any fluid loss from diarrhea by drinking more fluids and again, if it is chronic and not normal, talk to your doctor.

Now you can take out your blood pressure cuff. You should know your normal blood pressure, which should be less than 120 for the systolic, the top number and less than 80 on the diastolic, the lower number. High blood pressure is the silent killer, precursor of strokes and heart attacks. Be aware. But take your blood pressure in the morning before the stress of the day starts impacting those numbers. Sit quietly. Be sure you are not crossing your legs, talking, or thinking anxious thoughts. Be sure that your arm is at the level of your heart. If your blood pressure is a bit higher, simply note it down and keep track each morning. Is it consistently higher? Share these numbers with your doctor. Is your blood pressure higher than 180/120? Contact your doctor today. Blood pressure reflects how you feel and what you are thinking. If you are in pain or upset, your blood pressure will be higher than normal.

What is your pulse? Less than 100? Normal for you? Heart rate varies according to your activity, your stress level, your pain level. Heart rate gets higher with any stress, pain or activity. It also gets higher if you aren't drinking enough water. Any dizziness? Are you dehydrated? Lightheadedness may be from dehydration.

Feeling cold? Check your temperature. Is it higher than normal for you? If its greater than 99.6 it may indicate some kind of infection brewing. Your body is heating up to try to burn it off, speeding up your metabolism to produce more germ-killing white blood cells.

Next, step on the scale. Have you gained or lost weight? If you have some extra pounds on board and you notice some swelling in your ankles, you may have some fluid retention which would explain your increased shortness of breath. Do you need to ask about a diuretic or simply cut down on your salt? Salt holds water in your system. Too much salt along with a sluggish heart can lead to some congestive heart concerns with increasing fatigue and shortness of breath. Call your doctor.

Because your lungs are more fragile, they require a little bit of extra attention and maybe a little more love than your average bodily organ. Your lungs need to be protected from the invisible dangers that lurk behind every corner. An ounce of preparation and prevention can save a pound of problems. A cold for you can get a lot more serious than someone who doesn't have any lung disease.

Be aware of the early warning signs that might indicate a budding infection. The earlier that you identify them, the speedier that you can deal with them before they gain any momentum. Fever, sore throat, changes in the color or consistency of your phlegm, fatigue, and more shortness of breath than usual are indicators that it's time to call the office. Maybe you notice you are using your rescue inhaler more frequently. Maybe you are wheezing or coughing. Is your oxygen level lower than normal? Is your peak flow smaller than normal?

Recognize the red flags and call your doctor's office. Your doctor may prescribe some antibiotics and maybe some steroids to open you up and stop a brooding infection.

Chest tightness or a crushing pain is a red flag and may indicate a heart attack. If it doesn't ease with a few moments of rest, call 911. Do not delay.

Identify impending problems before they get worse. Being pro-active can save you from more serious exacerbations and hospitalizations. If you aren't sure, call. Your doctor's job is to be there for you when you need him, not just when you are healthy.

Patrick had been feeling exhausted. He had no stamina. When his blood was drawn for testing the tech asked him if he drank a lot of coffee. "It's just that your blood is the color of coffee. It's supposed to be bright red."

When he arrived home, there was a machine sitting in the floor of his living room. There were no attached instructions. On closer inspection, he understood it to be an oxygen concentrator and after calling and talking to the doctor he figured out how to operate it. But, even after using it, he still felt sludgy and further, began to experience throbbing headaches. "Oh, you need to put water in the humidifier. Breathing straight oxygen can dry out your sinuses." "Oh. Okay."

His headaches abated with the humidified oxygen, but his oxygen levels weren't improving. His doctor suggested he turn up the liter flow. Still, there was no change. After further study, his doctor finally recognized that Patrick did not have the inhalation power to trigger the concentrator to release the oxygen. Patrick needed a continuous flow. "That's why I can't take some of the inhaler medications," Patrick said. "It takes a strong in-breath to trigger the inhaler to release the medication. I lost some money on medicines I can't use, before we figured that one out."

Patrick obtained a continuous flow and his numbers improved, but they would drop with any exertion. After exploring options, Patrick found a cannula with flared nasal prongs allowing a larger flow. His oxygen stayed stable and Patrick was finally feeling more alive and animated. Things were improving.

"I realized quickly that if I wanted to be in the best condition I could be, I was going to have to learn everything I could about this disease. "COPD is about what you Can do," he said. "In the middle are Options, opportunities, and Persistence. Lastly, it's about what you Do not do."

When you are doing your daily self-assessment, expect to be healthy. Don't expect problems. But be realistic. You will have ups and downs. That is the challenge of life. Be ready if you fall, to trudge up the slope again.

Be prepared. A client at support group once announced that the most loving thing you can do for your family is to have all your paperwork, accounts, and passwords in a safe place accessible to those you love. Having a trust with powers of attorney and a living will spelled out makes your eventual departure less traumatic for those left behind. Everyone dies. Face it squarely and leave this gift behind. The woman had lost her husband recently and was confronted with the overwhelming problem of not knowing anything about his final wishes or any of his financial accounts. She had no access to his passwords and had no idea what they were. "He had always taken care of all the bills." Her sorrow at the loss of her husband was complicated with the frustration and anger of not knowing essential information regarding his wishes or his financial accounts.

Take a moment to write down your answers to these questions:

How well are you tuned into the evidence your body exhibits before problems occur?

_____

_____

_____

How promptly do you notify your physician when you encounter a potential problem?

_____

_____

_____

Would bringing a notebook to appointments help you keep track of information? How?

_____

_____

_____

How prepared are you if something should happen?

_____

_____

_____

25

Staying Healthy

"If you don't take time for your wellness you will be forced to make time for your illness." —J. Sunada

So, you have done your self-assessment and found that everything is within normal for you. How can you ensure that you stay that way? The most effective way is start with handwashing and hand sanitizing. Recent studies actually show that using a hand sanitizer can be more effective than handwashing, unless your hands are visibly dirty. You can have it conveniently in your pocket or purse when you are out and about. When should you use hand sanitizer? After touching anything that's not in your own home. Some clients are aware of the pen the secretary gives you to sign when you enter the office, the doorknobs, the TV remote when you are waiting in the lobby.

When out to a restaurant and using the restroom, wash your hands and turn off the water with your elbow if possible, Wave your hand to release the paper towel or use your elbow once again to push the lever, grab the paper towel, dry your hands and use the paper towel to open the door so that your clean hands are not touching the doorknob on your way out. Not everyone washes their hands as you may have guessed, but at least you walked out without carrying any new germs on you.

Keep your hands away from your face.

When coughing or sneezing, do it into your elbow, those germs will be further away from your hands so that you don't inadvertently infect others or re-infect yourself. We should all be like the people from India who greet each other with their hands folded together and a bow of their head; It's so much safer than shaking hands and picking up new germs. Shaking hands with others, then bringing your hands to your face and mouth is a common way to pick up an infection. Your level of alertness should be raised whenever you are out of your own home.

Keep your respiratory tract clean and clear. That includes good oral hygiene, brushing and flossing and regular checkups. It also includes clearing the phlegm from your throat. Phlegm can build up often at night while you are sleeping. It gets hard and crusty and can be difficult to remove. Not only can it block your airway but it can also be a nesting place for unwanted germs to grow. While you are still in the bathroom, take a glass of hot water, swallow it down and then do your huff-huff coughs (see below). the hot water moistens and warms the throat making it easier for you to remove the phlegm. Blowing into a flutter valve, a small device with a ping pong ball inside is a useful tool in pulling out stuck mucous. If you still have a problem, ask your doctor about a vibrating vest and ask your rehab team about percussion.

Huff Huff Coughs

Sit straight on the toilet, take a slow deep breath in, then exhale in spurts making a huff-huff sound as you exhale. Repeat this about three times till your throat and airway feel open and clear. Drinking lots of water will help keep your phlegm loose and your airway clear.

Stay healthy and avoid infection with these simple routines:

▶ Get enough sleep, walk daily and get your vaccines promptly.

▶ Avoid crowds; they harbor invisible germs.

▶ Don't offer to babysit the grandkids when they are sick. Kids transfer germs faster than anyone.

▶ Stay away from smokers. Avoid smoke and fireplaces. Instead of regular candles, use soy or electric candles.

▶ Make sure you change the air filter in your home every few months, don't forget to have the mechanic check your filter in your car as well.

▶ Be sure to have your car circulate your air so you are not taking in the exhaust from the cars in front of you while you are in traffic.

▶ Watch out for mold build up in your house, especially in those crevices in your bathroom, along the edge of the tub or shower. Black smudge that grows in the corners of your back closets or in the grout of your bathtub carry fungal spores. Fungus can find its way into your respiratory tract and begin to grow. Find a professional to eradicate it. Ask for a thorough inspection and cleaning if necessary.

▶ Plants can be wonderful air cleansers and oxygenate the air in your home but the soil can also carry mold. Apply some baking soda or a solution of water and apple cider vinegar, a natural antiseptic to your plants' soil. Keep rotting leaves out of the soil. These will help keep them free of mold.

Anything you can smell are tiny particles that are getting into your respiratory tract. Bleaches and ammonia cleaners are caustic to breathe. Soap and water is an effective tool against most virus and bacteria. Alcohol and hydrogen peroxide are effective disinfectants. Be sure to use gloves when cleaning and use according to directions. Never mix chemicals together. Try a fresh bouquet of flowers or maybe natural essential oils instead of air fresheners.

One night, the ambulance arrived at the ER where I was working and delivered a 45-year-old woman wearing an oxygen mask with an IV inserted in her arm. She apparently had been cleaning her bathroom at home when she suddenly felt her airway burn and tighten. She had dialed 911 and gasped out her address. She was in panic; her eyes were bulging as she struggled for air. We immediately injected some epinephrine and steroids, and gave nebulized bronchodilators. Within fifteen minutes she was breathing a little more easily but still painfully. She said that she had been scrubbing her bathroom appliances and had mixed some of the chemicals, bleach and ammonia together hoping to achieve a more thorough cleaning. Unfortunately, when she mixed these chemicals, poisonous fumes in the small airless room flowed into her respiratory tract and burned her airway. She stayed in the hospital for a few days until her airway improved and she was stable enough to go home. It was a difficult lesson to learn but one that I will always remember.

The chemicals that we store in our garage, in our cupboard, and use on our lawn can be deadly. If you suddenly have difficulty breathing or it becomes painful call 911. If you feel no symptoms but are concerned, call Poison Control. Poison Control is always available by phone. Don't wait. Poison Control will provide specific instructions on how to minimize the effects.

With a little thought and a little awareness, you can make your home and lifestyle as healthy and infection free as possible. You owe it to yourself to take your life and your health seriously. It's the most precious thing you have.

• • •

Take a moment to write down your answers to these questions:

What infection prevention strategies do you do in your daily routine?

_____

_____

_____

_____

What other strategies can you adopt to decrease your risk of infection?

_____

_____

_____

_____

Do you think that your state of mind affects your ability to resist infection? How?

_____

_____

_____

_____

26

Using Your Energy Wisely

"When you focus on problems, you'll have more problems. When you focus on possibilities, you'll have more opportunities." —Zig Ziglar

Energy is like money. You have a certain amount of it to use each day. And you don't want to squander it in the first few hours so that you have none left for later.

Before you get out of bed in the morning, take a few minutes to first, count your blessings, then create your day. This is going to be a great day! Decide right away. Having a mindset of positivity goes a long way to making your day as you plan. Remember, we always meet our expectations.

Plan: What is on the agenda for today? What tasks and errands do you need to accomplish today? What appointments and meetings are scheduled?

Prioritize: Prioritizing your tasks allows you to decide what you absolutely need to do today and what you could put off until tomorrow. Are some of these tasks those that can be delegated to family or friends or maybe be done by phone? When is your best energy? Is it in the morning? That is the time to carry out the important tasks, not later when your energy tends to wane.

Prepare: Luckily, you gave some thought to the day last night and set out your clothes, your lists, and your breakfast supplies so you can get up and get going quicker. Your keys are on the hook where they belong, easy to grab on the way out. Your inhalers are in the bathroom, laid out in order of short acting to long acting. Easy to self-administer. Great. Your grocery list is attached to your bag so you can stop at the store on your way back from your scheduled appointment.

The bathroom routine is organized. Maybe you take your short acting inhaler before showering. You keep the door and window open for extra air to circulate while you are showering so that the steam gets released quickly, the fan is on and the vent filter has been changed and is clean. There's a grab bar in the shower, and a seat for you to sit while showering. The oxygen tubing is long enough to easily wear while you are showering.

Position: You sit, lower your head and wash your hair, without having to raise your arms over your head. After showering, you grab your terrycloth robe and wrap it around you. You rest on the seat of the toilet and rest for a while. Your clothes are easily accessible from where you are sitting and you dress while sitting and slip into your loafer shoes.

Pace: You give yourself plenty of time, setting the alarm a half hour earlier so you don't have to rush. Rushing makes you short of breath which makes you anxious. When you get anxious, you get even more short of breath. Instead, you are methodical and mindful. There is no rushing. You stay relaxed, listening to your body, as you move from task to task.

Pursed lip breathing: You walk to the kitchen using your pursed lip breathing and find your stool. You sit. You grab the bowl and spoon from the counter that you have previously placed within reach from the stool.

Pause: You rest for a few minutes while you gather your thoughts, remembering to look outside and see the sky. You notice the birds chirping around the feeder outside. Taking a moment to collect your thoughts, you review the steps needed to get you on your way. By pausing, you become more mindful of what you are doing and more aware of the tasks at hand. You will be less likely to skip a step and have to backtrack. You will be less likely to make a mistake. "Pause for the cause," my hiker friend would say. Stay mindful.

Coffee on the counter is an arm's reach away and the cereal is in the lazy susan in the lower cabinet. You get up and grab the milk and fruit from the refrigerator and turn back to the bar where breakfast is waiting. Having an organized kitchen makes preparing meals and clean up so much easier and enjoyable.

You switch to your portable concentrator within reach and already in your roller. Taking a few relaxing pursed lip breaths and smiling, you saunter out to your garage, slide your concentrator into the car and slip into the driver's seat.

The journey of a thousand miles begins with one step. One step and you are closer to your destination. But if the step is a detour, the destination may become further away. Life's daily tasks can use a up a lot of your energy if not done wisely and efficiently. We all know the story of the race between the tortoise and the hare. The hare is quick and impulsive, expending lots of energy and exhausting himself. The tortoise is slow, steady, using his energy efficiently, moving towards the goal in a straight path.

Are you the tortoise or the hare? When the grocery clerk offers to help with bags, do you let him? If he doesn't, do you ask him?

When you get home, do you grab your dolly, placing the bags on the portable dolly and pull them into the house, or do you grapple with the bags exhausting yourself out?

A dolly helps with carrying groceries, carrying laundry, and pulling your portable concentrator, saving you energy to use on other worthwhile projects.

Instead of reaching up to grab the bowls on the top shelf, can you place them on a lower shelf for easier access or can you reach for the extended grabber? Your energy needs to be used for exercise and for walking on your terms.

• • •

Take a moment to write down your answers to these questions:

What part of your daily tasks consume the most energy?

_____

_____

_____

How can you better organize your time and your home?

_____

_____

_____

What tools and resources might be helpful in creating more efficiency?

_____

_____

_____

What actions can you take today?

_____

_____

_____

27

Researching All the Options

Thank you for helping to shape me into a person who now believes that anything is possible with love and endurance.

We live in an age in which information is easily accessible. It is up to you to remain up-to-date on the latest research studies, their conclusions, and what findings are confirmed or debunked. Studies related to lung disease are accessible on the web and the studies can be fascinating. Read the abstract, the summary of their project, and then scroll down to the discussion where you will find the results explained. Was the study successful? What were the parameters? What was the final conclusion? One study does not necessarily prove anything. It often only proves that there is room for further investigation. Review the information with your doctor and with the professionals in rehab. What is their take on it?

Jeremy had heard something about the ancient tradition of salt caves being helpful for lungs and he shared his findings with the group. "Well," I said, "the process of osmosis seems to support the idea of decreasing inflammation in the lungs." He told us about the effects on the workers in the salt mines. After checking it with Dr. Woods, he decided he would try it. Jeremy began getting regular weekly treatments in the salt room in the nearby city, finding relief and breathing easier.

Mel couldn't afford the salt room treatments but decided to try a salt lamp in her bedroom. She said she felt more open and she slept better.

Salt lamps have a history of helping people with respiratory issues as they clean the air of pollutants, they decrease the amount of negative electromagnetic energy from electrical devices. Some medical companies are even utilizing salt in their aerosolizers based on its positive effects on asthma and allergies. They may also help sleep and decrease anxiety.

Henry invested in an air purifier for his home. He said it made him feel more comfortable and maybe his breathing was easier. Air purifiers take out some of the dust, pollen, pet dander, and allergens.

If humidity bothers your breathing, a de-humidifier might be a good investment. If the dryness is more irritating, perhaps a humidifier might help. With any device, keeping it clean, changing filters regularly makes them function better and will avoid more problems.

Henry had biweekly visits with his chiropractor and had found that he felt better and had less bouts of sickness since starting biweekly treatments. Did you know that chiropractors can be helpful in alleviating the symptoms of COPD? A few studies have shown improvement in forced vital capacity, walking distance, and levels of dyspnea after chiropractic care.

Tai Chi improves breathing and respiratory function in COPD patients. It relieves stress and anxiety and strengthens respiratory muscles. Pulmonary function tests show improvement in studies of patients with COPD.

Short and spunky, Delores always had a kind word to share. She was like a mother to everyone. Delores faithfully went to Tai chi once a week. It's held at the senior center and its free. "You know, I used to get frequent colds and now, I just don't anymore. And my neuropathy in my feet is so much better than it was. I know it's because of the tai chi. I don't understand it, but I like doing it. Its relaxing." Peggy smiled and nodded.

Peggy had been attending pulmonary rehab for about eight years. When she first went to see Dr. Woods, she and her children had been shopping for caskets. Peggy and her family had thought that her life was coming to an end. That was back then. After starting pulmonary rehab, Peggy became too busy to spend time on that. Although preparations have been completed, she spent no time worrying about dying. She was too busy living. She organized the monthly lunches with the rehab gang, and checked up on those who missed class. She went to her tai chi classes on Monday with Delores and played Ma Jong with the girls on Wednesday.

Chinese complementary therapies are often based on the concept of energy channels throughout the body. Eastern Chinese medicine has proved itself through the centuries for non-acute health issues. Discuss complementary options with your physician first. Your pharmacist, and rehab team can also provide some insight and perspective.

Marge had heard about the successes of stem cell therapy and was eager to sign up. Her rehab team helped her better understand the current research and the promise of this new therapy. "Stem cell therapy for lung disease is still in its infancy and has not yet been shown to be that effective," Mary, the RN told her. "It is expensive too, and not covered by insurance. There's been some steps forward with spinal cord injuries and even with heart disease and diabetes. But these studies take years to complete and evaluate. Be patient though; I have faith that it might really be a possible future cure. But not yet. Other therapies are less expensive and can also help you feel better."

Some pulmonary rehab programs are fortunate enough to have a reiki therapist provide treatments to patients during their rehab sessions. Initial research on the effectiveness of Reiki in pulmonary disease showed increased ease of breathing and decreased discomfort. It is noninvasive and calming. Many have found reiki to be relaxing, allowing them to breathe easier and sleep better at night.

Herbal supplements can be helpful for decreasing phlegm and opening airways. Be sure to check in with the pharmacist and doctor before exploring these supplements. Breathe easy tea was a favorite. N-acetylcysteine (NAC) can be effective in breaking up mucous, which can be a big problem for many. Cayenne in safe doses may help open up sinuses and airways.

Cordyceps is a Chinese herb that has been traditionally used to treat lung disease. Some studies find that it appears to have some positive effects, though these studies are limited. Vitamin C is an immune enhancer and may prevent exacerbations. Taking immune support tablets might help fight off potential infections.

Monolaurin is an herb that has anti-viral, anti-fungal, and anti-bacterial qualities. It is used to keep our livestock and poultry healthy. It might have a similar effect on humans. Ginger is an antiviral herb which, when used as a chest rub, can help bring up mucous. Curcumin (Turmeric) has been shown to decrease the inflammation in your bronchial tree that leads to tightness and shortness of breath. Check in first with your doctor and pharmacist before starting any supplement program. Remember, even supplements, in conjunction with some meds, can be toxic.

Acupuncture is a traditional Chinese treatment in which tiny needles are gently and painlessly inserted into your skin at various points related to the energy channels in your body. By stimulating these channels, energy is allowed to flow more easily into the areas needing it. It may help improve breathing and stamina.

Massage therapy may be beneficial in improving pulmonary function.

Practicing expanding and constricting your lungs and chest wall by playing a harmonica, or a kazoo, or even singing, can help your breathing. Singing and playing music also increases serotonin levels, making you more relaxed and feeling good all over.

These are complementary therapies which means they work best in conjunction with your medications, not by themselves.

Martha is a 40-year-old woman with so much vibrant energy, her body simply didn't comply with her personality. But she was steadfast in her exercise program. Maintaining her oxygen levels in the low 90's to upper 80's and challenging her fatigued muscles to do a little more and a little more. Despite her efforts her lungs were deteriorating quickly. Martha was a positive one, though. She would arrive with a laugh and show immense appreciation for rehab, for her good fortune and health. She boosted the morale of the others on difficult days, sharing stories and listening to their concerns. "Being courageous is not about doing an amazing task, single-handedly," she'd say. 'It's about facing whatever it is, and helping others over their obstacles at the same time. We are a team!" Healthy, except for her lungs, it was time to talk about a transplant. She had met and chatted with some of our other clients who had gone through the procedure and decided that a transplant would be right for her. They reminded her that the tests were worse than the procedure, but each one she met confirmed that they were glad that they did it.

Life before, during, and after transplant is not easy and you must pass multiple tests, some physical and some psychological. It's not a cure all but a trade-off. It restricts you to frequent monitoring at the pulmonary center and expectations that you religiously follow through on self-administering multiple medications on a daily basis. It's not without risk. The medication all come with side effects including decreasing your ability to recognize and fight off invading infectious germs.

Martha successfully received a transplant, and recently returned from a sporting competition in Europe, a champion, glowing with joy. "With my new lungs, I still get it that life is lived one moment at a time..."

. . .

Take a moment to write down your answers to these questions:

How open are you to trying new strategies and treatments?

_____

_____

_____

_____

What do you have the most difficulty with and how can you find a solution?

_____

_____

_____

_____

What have you found to be helpful that you might share with others?

_____

_____

_____

_____

28

Have Fun, Believe in Yourself!

"Great things never come from comfort zones." —B. Francia

It's hard to be depressed when you are surrounded by friends, enjoying things you love to do. Even though fatigue may have caused you to slow down, continue to be outgoing and social when you have the energy. It's okay if you don't make every meeting or every outing. Others will appreciate you even more when you do make it!

Move out of your comfort zone! That's how we grow! Join the club! Any club! Be part of a fun and rewarding experience once a week. Find your passion: Bridge, games, book clubs, libraries, senior centers, drawing, writing, or movie groups, pool room competitions, or church gatherings.

Someone a few years ago, started a program called meetup.com. And wherever you live now, there are groups run by people like you who are looking to create a group experience in wherever their interests lie. Look it up.

If you are fortunate enough to be 50 or older you can access all the wonderful events at the senior center. So many vibrant and happy people arrive to take part in an amazing array of activities. They are usually free or pretty darn cheap. The local community college may have opportunities to learn and grow and share. Stretch yourself!

Yes, you have those days when getting out of bed in the morning takes more effort. Accept it, enjoy the movie marathon and be gentle with yourself for a day. Just know when to get back into the saddle. The more frequently you allow yourself to sit out, the harder it gets to jump back up again. Don't find yourself in the pit, unable to move. Be brave. If you know once you up and out, you will be fine, push a little and get out. If you slack off for long, you will lose more energy and start sinking.

Mothers of young children are not allowed to be sick or incapacitated as their children need to be cared for every day. So, they do it. Sometimes that pressure of being needed has that positive effect. Corrinne never missed a day of work. She couldn't afford to. It's what she did. This doesn't mean that you are the same way.

Feelings are a big part of you, feel them but don't swallow them. Have a pity party.... for fifteen minutes at a specified time. No longer. Not before, not after. Then, move on...you'll find that in a short while you will forget to take those fifteen minutes. Don't hang on to resentments, grief, regrets, and guilt. No one is perfect. We are all just learning and practicing the game of life here and we all make so many mistakes at it. Let it go, forgive yourself, and the others, and move on.

Start the day with a breath, a stretch, and a smile and finish it by remembering the best parts of your day. For me, the best parts of my day are always the ones where I am sharing with others. For others, it may be checking 'done' on your to do list. Whatever it is, give back and share your gifts.

Laugh. An editor of a large NY firm, Norman Cousins, was diagnosed with ankylosing spondylitis, a painful progressive disease. Prescribed treatments were ineffective and caused further physical risks and problems. Norman took the reins, deciding that he would cure himself. He would stay positive, watching funny movies for several hours every day and take large quantities of vitamin C. Mr. Cousins overcame his illness, and in the process, discovered what is now known as 'psychoneuroimmunology', the study of the effects of the mind on the body. It is true, 'laughter is the best medicine'! By improving his state of mind, his body was able to recover on its own. He wrote a bestselling book, *Anatomy of An Illness*.

The author of chicken soup for the soul taped a plastic million-dollar bill to his ceiling so that each morning when he woke, it would be the first thing he saw. And he would be reminded that this is what he would achieve within the year. He was living hand to mouth at this stage, hoping that his book would find a publisher. After 44 publisher rejections and 14 months later, he found his publisher. He did not reach his goal of making a million that year, He earned only $999,900.00. But if he hadn't had that reminder each morning, how much would he have made?

So, tape your goal to the ceiling above your bed so that you are reminded each morning. Stick it on your refrigerator so that each time you open the door, it's in your vision. 'I am breathing easy'. 'My lungs are getting better every day, and in every way'. 'I am healthy and energized!' 'I am playing golf.' 'I am riding my bike!' See it, believe it!

Sun Yeong arrived with her two grown children at the rehab center for her initial assessment. She had recently been discharged from the hospital after a long bout with pneumonia. She was a little woman but fiercely determined. Her expression was strong and serious. When it was time for her six-minute walk, Sun Yeong could not stand up from her wheelchair. She pushed with her arms again and again but after almost a month of recuperating she had no strength left. At the time, patients who could not stand and transfer to a machine independently were not allowed into the program. With sadness, Sandy confessed to her that she was not a candidate for pulmonary rehab. "We must do something," the children said. "How can she improve?" Sandy taught them to assist their mother to a standing position, and placing a pillow on her seat, set her back down. Repeat this process again and again until she needs only one-sided assistance, then, continue until she can do it alone. Once she can do it alone, walk with her two steps maybe three steps at a time and help her sit down. Make sure she has a good high protein diet. "Here are some stretch bands for her to use to strengthen her legs and her arms."

Sun Yeung returned in two weeks to try again. She had practiced every day, she said in her broken English, and she wanted to try again. Sandy was already impressed with her persistence but when she returned, she independently transferred herself with noticeable effort, to the recumbent machine. Then, she walked several steps for 4 seconds with some assistance. This little lady, who two weeks ago could not stand up from her wheelchair had come so far! Clapping her hands in joy, Sandy welcomed her to the program with the understanding that her exercise homework continue. Sun Yeung continued to grow stronger and stronger. Her daughter brought her each day and watched her exercise. A quiet little lady, she said little but always had a smile. She was always eager to push herself more. Sun Yeung's strength and stamina grew with each passing week and she soon transferred from wheelchair to monitored walks and finally, the treadmill. She started using the treadmill for one minute, then two as the team monitored her breathing and oxygen levels.

On her fifteenth session Sun Yeong arrived without her wheelchair. She was using her walker. From the parking lot to

Pulmonary Rehab on the second floor was a good four-minute walk. The team cheered when she walked into the gym. Everyone was so proud of her and so impressed. With determination and support, she became, once again, an interdependent, contributing member of her family and she was very proud. On her final rehab session, she arrived with homemade pastry to share with everyone. It was delicious. "I made it myself!" She said, proudly.

The irony is that, like Sun Yeong, many of these pulmonary heroes attribute their achievements to the therapists and nurses in outpatient rehab. But they are simply the coaches. Sun Yeong accomplished her goals because she worked at it. She made the decision and followed it through to her goal. Her family, friends and her team simply believed in her and helped her through. She was a hero.

There are lots of unexplained cures. We have all heard of situations where tumors have vanished and cancers have disappeared. Since these cases do not fit the criteria required for medical journals and cannot be explained scientifically, they are swept under the rug, never to be tabulated or investigated. The key is that they believed in themselves and in their own power to heal. How much of our health is subconscious? Ah, again the amazing unrecognized healing ability of our own body.

There was a famous case of a wealthy businessman who was severely injured in a plane crash and barely survived. The several physicians that he consulted with were all sure that he would never walk again. A new drug was introduced for study on the market which claimed to be a miracle cure. The man signed up. In three months' time he was walking out of the hospital on his own. He returned to his life as a vibrant and adventurous businessman, appreciative of this opportunity this wonderful drug was giving him. Two years later, he read in the papers that the drug he had taken was a failure. The studies proved that it did not work at all. Within a month this man was again unable to walk, he deteriorated rapidly until he finally passed away. It seemed that his belief in the drug was strong enough to cure him. When he stopped believing he succumbed.

Expect to feel better.

Expect that your medications are healing you.

Appreciate all you have. Even on the tough days.

When driving, each red light you come to is a reminder for you to count your blessings.

Before sleeping each night recall the three best things that happened during that particular day and fall asleep remembering them.

Expect miracles. Every day! My friend, Henry looked each day for those miracles and invariably each day, most often before noon, he discovered them. Watch for them.

Tell them that you love them. As often as you can. You know who they are. That includes yourself. Love yourself, be gentle, appreciate, and never underestimate your body's resiliency to heal.

Life is a gift. Life is a dynamic and ever-changing experience. The one thing you can bet on is that life will change. Learn to adapt to change, flow with it without trying to grab hold against the current. That can be exhausting and fruitless. The current of a river winds through the trees and ripples over rocks in its bed. Live your life like the river. Understand that there are rocks but keep flowing. If a river stops flowing, it stagnates.

A vehicle with a full tank of gas is ready for the journey. If it has no destination, it ends up in the same place. Have a destination.

Take time to notice the birds. Watch the sunrise.

'As I gaze over the skyline in the city, I marvel at all the creations of man. But none is so complex and as amazing as life itself.'

Being well doesn't mean that your body functions perfectly. No one's body functions perfectly. And muscle does not grow in a day. Just like in golf, everyone in this life has a handicap; some are noticeable, most are not. And often, if we can see the baggage that other people carry, we are most likely to pick up our own and feel lucky.

There will be failures and disappointments. Applaud yourself, first, for trying. No one ever failed who did not try....and see each failure and disappointment as a teacher. What can you learn from this and how can you use it to make life better for yourself and others?

Frank was a retired engineer. He had been a navy seal when he was younger and would relay stories of his adventures, jumping from airplanes, swimming through shark infested waters, and rappelling down buildings. He came to rehab and really loved the exercise. He seemed to do better and better. Frank connected easily and quickly with the other clients, sharing anecdotes and stories. Suddenly, Frank was missing from class and the team was concerned. We called and found that he had suffered an exacerbation and was in the hospital. We all missed him and someone called to check up on him every week. When Frank returned, he was carrying his oxygen, moving a lot slower. He had lost a lot of weight. Despite it all, he smiled and said he was ready to start over. When we age, we lose muscle mass very quickly when we don't maintain steady exercise and movement.

Fatigue, then shortness of breath sets in making it harder to move. But Frank was determined. He said it was the navy seal in him that just wouldn't allow self-pity or failure. Frank began again, moving at a slow pace on the nu-step and gradually he built up to the treadmill once again. His smile never wavered; his sense of confidence stayed strong. "Setbacks happen," he says. The key is to just get up again and go from there.

Steve doesn't get out too much these days but each day he remembers to prepare an ice cold bottle of water for the postal worker in the summer. "She is always so happy to see me. I see her coming with the mail and I get it out of the freezer. Its hot out there. It makes her day a little easier and she is so grateful. My advice to people like me: focus on the needs of others rather than yourself."

You are a hero. You have already accomplished so much and now you face a new challenge. Remember your accomplishments, your creations, your strengths, and feel good about them. Remember all those who helped you achieve. That's what will give you the stamina and the motivation to achieve success again. It's not just about discovering that hero inside you. By doing this you motivate others to become their own heroes. And that's the best thing of all.

Happiness is a state of mind. And what we think is what we find.

I am not a specialist in curing or treating lung disease. I am the nurse who greets you each morning in rehab, asks you how you are feeling, encourages and listens to you.

And what matters after all? Doing what we can for others. You know, the others who are doing less than you. And yes, there are always those who are doing so much less than you and they need your support. Be a hero for them.

• • •

Take a moment to consider your answers to these questions?

What is the most important thing you have learned?

_____

_____

_____

_____

What have you done so far to improve?

_____

_____

_____

_____

What are your next steps?

_____

_____

_____

_____

29

Joe: Reinventing A New and Better Life

*"I am not what happened to me but what I choose to become." —*M. Mcullum

Last week, Joe and Ellie started taking walks in the morning to the park. It was early spring and the weather was sunny and warm. Joe had gained back some weight and his six-foot two frame had some of his old muscle definition back. He was starting to look and act like himself again, Ellie observed. They held hands and meandered down to the pond. There, they settled on the bench, watching the ducks and the occasional heron. He would have never imagined that this would ever be possible again and yet, here they were. "I reached my goals, Ell." He sighed, as he placed his oxygen pack on the bench next to him, a look of contentment on his face. "Time for a new one then, Joe. We can talk about the next one on your list." Joe scanned the horizon, recalling the past eight months. Joe had thought that he was dying a slow horrible death. And here he was, feeling the sun on his face, looking at the girl he fell in love with.

"Did I ever tell you what happened to Humpty Dumpty after he fell? Well, old Humpty picked himself back up, put himself back together the best he could and started climbing. He was deathly afraid of heights, but he decided that he just wouldn't look down; he'd just keep looking up." He laughed. That same laugh that Ell had fallen in love with when they got married and she smiled. "And you know what happened when he reached the top? Joe smiled, "His shell cracked open"; Joe paused, "and he turned into a bird and he flew away."

"You've climbed a long way up from that pit. Don't make me say, 'I told you so', but you have guts, Joe, and you don't give up; you pulled through, just like you did that time we hit that snowstorm in Colorado, remember? I knew you wouldn't give up."

"I'm not the same man I was before, Ell." "I know, Joe, you're better" she laughed, "and funnier!" Ellie's eyes sparkled; her blonde hair fluttered in the breeze. Joe suddenly felt like the infatuated kid who couldn't keep his eyes off his bride.

The dour advice from that hospitalist when they discharged him was maybe taken way out of proportion. At his last appointment, his pulmonologist had mentioned that he was doing great, just as he had expected.

"I just had to redesign a few things in my life, learn a few lessons, I guess. I can think of easier ways to learn them but that's life. When you think it's going to be a home run, you suddenly get slammed on first base." He said, shaking his head, remembering. He remembered how exhausted he had felt, back then, and how much effort it took to pull himself up out of that lazy boy. Things changed; so had he.

"I feel much more alive in some ways than I ever did. I spent so much time at work I forgot to live life. And all the time it was always here, the things I didn't notice or take time to see. The important things end up being the little moments, like now, I notice how beautiful you are. I love walking with you in the mornings, the feel of the sun on my face. I love watching the hummingbirds with you at the breakfast table and helping with the cooking. I never realized that I could be such a good cook or that I would enjoy it so much. I like having coffee at Starbucks on Wednesday with the guys, solving all the world's problems. I like being able to help out with the support group."

Ellie, listened, looking into Joe's eyes, seeing those rays of wisdom dawn on him like a rainbow after a storm.

"Should have retired years ago," he said, "We've had enough money. Guess it's easy to simply do what you've always done; maybe because you just don't know how to do anything else. I sure wouldn't wish this on anyone; but for me it jolted me into what really matters in life.

There will always be another challenge down the road, I know, but each time I get over the hurdle, I get stronger, strong enough to handle the next one.

"And besides, today is perfect, I just want to enjoy it….and remember it forever. I love you, Ellie. Thank you for sticking by me even when I was a sludge." He leaned over and kissed her, stretching his arm around her back, pulling her closer. "I love you, Joe. I always will. And I sure do love the wonderful coffee you make for me every morning." Ellie laughed.

Ellie remembered back; she had been a little nervous, well, a lot nervous there for a while, wondering if he would really pull through it. But life has a way of giving us curve balls when we are least expecting them. And Joe had hit that curve ball and had made it to first base. She was proud of him; she felt closer to him now than she had in years.

"It's a trade-off, not having the stamina to play golf or run anymore but I've always wanted to get back into playing the drums and I've been thinking of getting one of those electric sets." Joe had connected with some of the guys in rehab and sometimes they went out to lunch after their session. "One of the guys, you know, Brett, remember him? Brett had played in a band back in college. He said he was a mean lead in the 70's, doing solos like Eric Clapton and he's getting back into playing again. I know it's been a while since I played the drums. That was before the kids." Joe's eyes scanned the horizon, thinking. "Brad thought maybe we could put something together. Might be fun." Ellie's face lit up. "That sounds exciting, Joe! This could be your next goal!"

"Actually, my next goal is to take that cruise with you to Hawaii." He chuckled, "There's a cruise ship called 'Sea Puffers' and they have oxygen supplies and respiratory therapists on board to help if we need it. There's one heading out this September and I put a down payment on it." Joe had a roguish smirk on his face. "I wanted to surprise you." "Oh, Joe!" Tears welled up in Ellie's eyes as her hand flew to her mouth in surprise. She then flung her arms around him and laughed so hard, the tears streamed down her face. "You will never cease to amaze me!"

You never know where tomorrow will lead you. All you have is today. That's why they call it the present; it is truly a gift. Dream, but don't forget to notice this present. Life is lots of little moments. Be good to yourself. Try new things, stretch beyond your comfort zone. Have fun. Be a hero.

• • •

If you change yourself, you will change your world.

—Mahatma Gandhi

30

COVID-19: Prevention - Survival - Recuperation

Jack got off the plane and headed for baggage claim. It had been a long quiet week, visiting with family in Chicago, as restaurants bars and all other forms of entertainment had been shut down due to this virus thing. He felt exhausted. Good to be home, he thought as he grabbed his luggage and headed for the Uber stand.

Two days later, his throat burned, and his body felt like he had doubled his workout at the gym; every muscle was groaning. Probably picked up a cold on the flight home, he assumed. He had been sleeping for the past 16 hours. Unusual for him but he chalked it up to the long flight and the exhaustion from dealing with family all week. Today was the presentation in front of the board. He couldn't be late; his team was waiting for him.

COVID-19. Corona Virus Disease 2019. Invisible, highly contagious, sinister, deadly for many. It chooses its targets like a roulette game. One experiences a few days of queasiness and fatigue. Another becomes incapacitated, hospitalized, attached to a ventilator in intensive care, battling for his life. And still another remains symptom free yet COVID-19 positive and infectious after exposure. Initially considered a threat to older people, there are increasing percentages of people under 65 hospitalized and suffering with COVID-19. If you have other health issues including lung disease, cancer, diabetes, high blood pressure, or immunosuppression, your risk of infection is greater.

In early 2020, South Korea was able to control the spread of the virus with quarantine, mask wearing, testing and tracing. The virus had seemingly been abolished. One evening soon after, a 29-year-old gentleman arrived in Seoul, the capital of South Korea and visited five bars in one evening. The following week, eighty people were identified as COVID-19 positive. Those, in turn, infected their communities and the pandemic erupted full force once again.

SARS-CoV-2 is the official name of the virus that causes the disease known as COVID-19. It is a member of a very large family of viral diseases with well-known relatives, like SARS (Severe Acute Respiratory Syndrome of 2003) and MERS (Middle East Respiratory Syndrome of 2012). Each member of the family has common characteristics yet each are more or less virulent and contagious. COVID-19 is wrapping its tendrils around the entire world. Compared to the flu, mortality rate is significantly higher.

COVID-19 was first found to be spreading rapidly in late 2019, throughout the population around Wuhan, China, a huge metropolis. International travel and normal socialization escalated the spread of the pandemic. At this point in time, every part of the world is working to control this virus.

The virus primarily invades humans via droplets, moisturized air from an infected human carrier. In 2 to 14 days, shortness of breath, sore throat, cough, fever, and fatigue strike like a bolt of lightning and you are a statistic. Older people may have gastrointestinal symptoms or none at all except for a diminishing blood oxygen level.

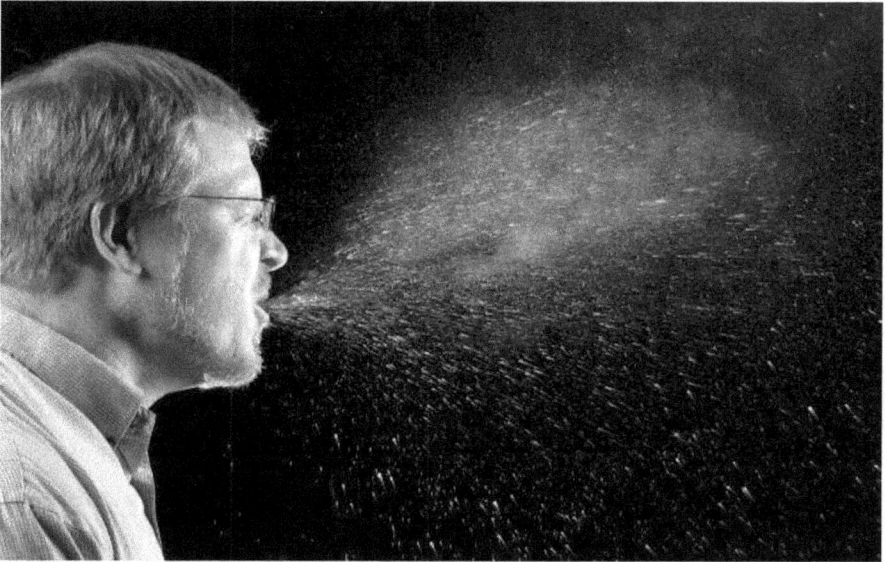

What does that mean for you? Dr. Chin Hong, Infectious Disease Specialist explains it as "The three W's to ward off COVID-19: wearing a mask, washing your hands, and watching your distance." Because there are so many asymptomatic carriers of the disease (Those who are COVID-19 positive but have no symptoms), you can't tell who is infected.

Always, always wear a mask while outside the home. If you have access to a surgical mask, or an N-95, it may be more effective in keeping you safe. Wearing a cloth mask will help to keep others safe while providing some personal protection. The mask should cover your nose and mouth to be effective. Masks with one-way valves may provide you with some protection but it is not effective in protecting others.

Protective eyewear should also be considered as a recent study funded by WHO shows evidence of transmission via the eye.

Do masks really work? A man flew from China to Toronto and subsequently tested positive for COVID-19. He had a dry cough and wore a mask on the flight, and all 25 people closest to him on the flight tested negative for COVID-19. In another case, in late May, two hair stylists in Missouri had close contact with 140 clients while sick with COVID-19. Everyone wore a mask and none of the clients tested positive.

In an analysis of data on transmission of the virus in June of 2020, scientists predicted that if 95% of people wore masks 95% of the time while out in public, infection rates would be cut in half.

Physical distancing is also a priority. Remaining at home with family as much as is possible prevents exposure to infection. Limiting other social interaction to phone calls, online connections and posts allow you to stay connected with friends and loved ones safely. Be sure to write cards and make those phone calls each day just to check in. Avoid restaurants and bars.

While working with public health, educating health care workers on infection control in long term care facilities, I emphasized the need for prevention protocols not only while working with their patients but also on their break. Eating and drinking is impossible while wearing a mask. Yet, eating and drinking exacerbates the spread of droplets. When you talk across the table to your friends and colleagues while eating, you share much more than conversation. Simply be sure to sit at least six feet from each other, especially at lunchtime.

You can still get out and walk if the weather permits. Unless specific local rules are prohibiting it, going outside and taking a walk where you stay at least 6 feet away from others can be a great, safe way to stay healthy. Staying flexible and strong can make a huge difference in your resilience and resistance to the virus. Review chapter 20 on strategies you can do at home.

Try doing some daily breathing exercises as outlined in chapter 14. Stretch the lungs each day for five minutes, expanding and contracting deeply and fully. The chi gong breath and the yogic jar breathing techniques may improve lung capacity and resilience. Stretch your arms up over your head, while lying on your back and feel your diaphragm expand.

If it is necessary for you to venture into public places like supermarkets or shops, or in areas where you will run across other people, avoid getting closer than six feet to anyone, and always be wearing your mask. In crowded public places, the virus floats in the air dropping down towards new victims. Avoid the crowds. Check with the store clerk to find out what day and time the store is least busy. That is when you might plan your shopping. Wash your hands when you return home.

Contracting the virus from contaminated surfaces is possible. An infected person handles a surface before you arrive, then you handle the surface, you maybe touch your face or mouth infecting yourself with the virus.
Wash your hands for twenty seconds after handling materials from outside the home and use hand sanitizer frequently while out.

Disinfecting surfaces like doorknobs, TV remotes, light switches, packages with bleach solution, soap and water or alcohol will kill the virus. Do not ingest any chemical not approved by your doctor.

Thanks to the unrelenting efforts of virologists and infectious disease specialists, Remdesivir and other related medications are showing success in improving the outcome for many of those infected. Virologists have created vaccines which are in the process of large-scale testing for efficacy.

There appears, at this time, to be several nonfactual and harmful theories being circulated through social media. Verify the source of any information you receive about the virus or its transmission. Be sure the information coincides with the CDC, WHO and Public Health offices.

In the meantime, people young and old continue to get sick. "I wouldn't wish this on anyone; it's horrible." Stacey, recuperating these past three weeks along with her husband and two young children is not sure where they may have been exposed to the virus but considers that it may have occurred during their recent travel out of state. "And when you do finally recuperate" Stacey continues, her voice cracking as she tries to stifle the tears, "I worry that there may be residual complications to the heart or the lungs. Of course, we are young and healthy but not knowing if my husband or my children will suffer long term health problems is devastating." Worry and fear exacerbate the overwhelming exhaustion she feels.

Donald and Norma were heading back from a vacation in New Zealand just as COVID-19 was invading the US in March of 2020. Transferring flights in LA, they were both escorted to an assigned CDC assessment room where a large group of vacationers from Italy were assembled waiting to be tested. After a few hours, they were finally released to resume their journey back home. "That's where I picked up the infection," said Donald, "packed in that room with all the tourists returning from Italy." Italy's infection rates, at that very same time, were skyrocketing.

Finally home, Donald returned to work the following day. Four days later, he was admitted to the hospital, and in another 24 hours, he was in the ICU on a ventilator. 72 years old, active and healthy except for his high blood pressure, Donald was in the hospital for 28 days and in extended care for another three weeks. "I don't remember anything until a few days before I was discharged to extended care. I remember I tried to put my glasses on but couldn't grab them. I couldn't pick up a spoon." He had lost all his fine motor function. "This won't last," he thought to himself, "Ill get better at this."

Norma, meanwhile, not allowed to see her husband or even communicate with him, waited for the daily check in call from the doctor. On the sixth day, the doctor called her and said "He is still critical but stable...ummmm, yes, he's day six. It's usually the seventh day that we lose them..." Norma erupted, "Please, from now on call my son, not me."

Not being there with him was the hardest part. "Every patient in a hospital needs an advocate, someone to watch over what happens, making sure that they get the care they need and I wasn't allowed in."

Donald returned home without any complications. He used his walker for the first few days and then he walked. He developed a routine of exercises and walking, each day pushing a little more. After another month he was back playing golf and helping his son renovate his home.

"What I would advise is that people have a thermometer and an oximeter at home. Monitor your temperature and your oxygen daily. A rising temperature will indicate that you are getting sick with the virus. And oxygen levels can drop rapidly. If they start dropping, get yourself to the hospital."

Conquering the COVID-19 virus can be exhausting and may have taken all your stamina, all your effort. Many are not as lucky as Donald and recover only to confront a new set of challenges. How you continue to navigate through this depends on you.

Some people return to normal functioning after weeks or months of recuperation, while others have permanent scarring. Because of the massive inflammatory response to the virus, many are left to cope with damage to their lungs, requiring long term oxygen therapy. Continued cough, shortness of breath, fatigue and the need for oxygen may be due to Post COVID-19 Fibrosis.

Look at the positives first! You are alive and back with your family, your wife, your parents, your kids. You can laugh, enjoy ice cream and watch the clouds sail across the sky. Be grateful and notice that its all the tiny moments in life that matter most. But what is next? How do you put yourself back together?

Remember, after several weeks in bed, muscles shrink, digestive processes slow, heart and blood vessels weaken, thoughts become skewed. It takes time to rebuild.

Donald explained how he did it. "My philosophy during this whole thing and even before, was that if you can change something, change it. If you can't, live with it."

Don't allow yourself to vegetate, move forward. One step at a time. Where do you want to be? Where are you now? Be gentle with yourself and find your support, your resources. Your doctor can connect you to therapies and groups. You are not alone. There are now and may well be thousands more going through this transition. Utilize your experience, your skills to adapt and adjust.

Open your mind to new perspectives. Consider options. Creating a realistic plan with specific objectives and a timeline may focus your attention and spur you into action. Focused action towards your objective brings you closer. And with each success, reward yourself.

Find valid online sites that can direct you towards getting post COVID-19 advice. Sue found satisfaction in creating a post COVID-19 recuperation group on Facebook to help support and encourage others like her.

Like Sue, find what brings you joy and satisfaction.

To improve your health and your lungs be sure to carry out breathing exercises daily, exploring the capacity of your lungs without causing pain. Just as with other exercises, the more you do the more you can do. You may find that happening as you monitor your incentive spirometer or your peak flow meter.

Move. As discussed in chapter 20, don't succumb to your feeling of exhaustion. The less you do, the less you feel like doing. I am not encouraging a full-blown work out but create a schedule and a plan in which you can move for a certain number of minutes a day. Break it up to 5 minutes each 3 hours of the day. Dance, walk, sit stand, sway and swing, lift some soup cans up and down, simply move. Yes, you feel you have no energy. Use what energy you have to move your muscles. Any muscles. Stretch and constrict each muscle, from your toes all the way up to your scalp.

Engage your mind in things outside yourself. Find a way to express, support, share with those who need it. You'll find that the currency of energy returns fourfold to you. Maybe its through a face book support group, a book club or a newspaper article. Share your experience. Others can learn from you. You have so much to share. Get out of yourself.

Keep alert to the studies being reported. Focus on the abstract and discern the point of the study and the results. Then, discuss with your doctor. Is there something that might help you? This is a learning process for you as well the scientists and doctors. Vital information is released daily. You must be your own advocate in your own life, your own prognosis. It's not what the doctor or the journalist says that is most important, but what you tell yourself.

Life brings change and challenge. With each challenge you overcome, you are stronger and better. With each change you become more flexible, and more understanding of others. It could be worse; it could always be worse. So count your blessings, rest up, and then, move forward. One step at a time. Open your heart and mind to the possibilities.

About the Author

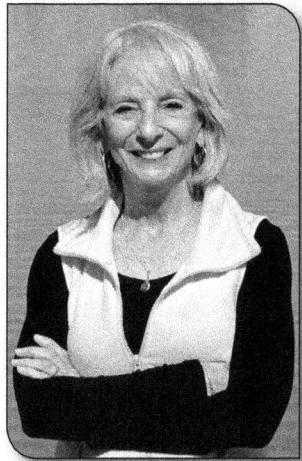

Photo by Carley Barton

A nurse and a health educator, Marilyn Klingler RN, B.S., M.Ed. has practiced nursing for 40 years in several specialties including intensive care, emergency, cardiac and pulmonary specialties. Her true passion is in Pulmonary Rehab where she has learned so much more from her patients than from her medical books. Marilyn has presented on strategies for better outcomes for pulmonary patients at the AZ State Nurses Association Annual Conferences, and at the State and National Cardiac and Pulmonary Rehab Association Annual Conferences. She has given presentations at hospital and community groups throughout AZ. Winner of the American Association of Cardiovascular and Pulmonary Rehab Innovation Award, she continues to explore new and better avenues to improve the health and wellness of the pulmonary population.

PARTNERING FOR BRONCHIECTASIS SOLUTIONS

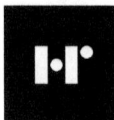

Hillrom™

Often masked by other lung conditions, such as COPD and asthma, bronchiectasis (BE) is more common than you may realize.[1] Early intervention, with treatments that can include antibiotics, medications and airway clearance therapy, is key to slowing BE progression.

Let's work together to increase awareness of BE. Visit LivingWithBE.com for helpful patient and clinician resources.

hillrom.com

1. Seifer F, Hansen G and Weycker D. Health-care utilization and expenditures among patients with comorbid bronchiectasis and chronic obstructive pulmonary disease in US clinical practice. Chron Respir Dis 2019: Jan-Dec;16. doi: 10.1177/1479973119839961

The Vest® is a registered trademark of Hill-Rom Services PTE Ltd. Hill-Rom reserves the right to make changes without notice in design, specifications and models. The only warranty Hill-Rom makes is the express written warranty extended on the sale or rental of its products.

© 2020 Hill-Rom Services PTE Ltd. ALL RIGHTS RESERVED. APR108601 rev 1 29-JUN-2020 ENG – US